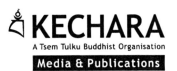

MRCP II
(INTERNAL MEDICINE)
MADE EASY

W.M.Chong

Kechara Media & Publications Sdn Bhd
2009

Kechara Media & Publications Sdn Bhd
5-2, Jalan PJU 1/3G
SunwayMas Commercial Centre
47301 Petaling Jaya
Selangor, Malaysia

TEL: [+603] 7805 5691
FAX: [+603] 7805 5690
EMAIL: kmp@kechara.com
WEBSITE: www.kechara.com/kmp

The moral right of the author has been asserted.

ISBN 978-967-5365-01-0

COVER AND BOOK DESIGN:
Jeannie Chen / Knottyforest Creative

PRINTED BY:
Pony Prints (M) Sdn Bhd
No. 41 & 43, Jalan Jasa Merdeka 1A
Taman Datuk Tamby Chik Karim
Batu Berendam
75350 Melaka
Malaysia

TEL: [+606]-3178328
FAX: [+606]-3178327

CONTENTS

FOREWORD

From the few encounters I have had with Dr. Chong and from what people have observed, I have found him to be extremely kind and generous, and a very dedicated person in his profession. Being a doctor is one of the most beneficial careers that we can have; being a dedicated doctor who has deep concern for his patients makes this person stand out and even more beneficial.

Within our Kechara Buddhist organisation in Malaysia, we have a department for community work, known as Kechara Soup Kitchen. Dr. Chong has gone out on their weekly rounds to offer food to the homeless many times. Not only does Dr. Chong participate in giving nourishment to the urban poor of Kuala Lumpur, he also takes the time to talk to these people, diagnoses any medical problems they may have and even treats them on the spot. This has been observed by our volunteers many times, and is a clear indication he is a very caring and dedicated doctor.

The publication of this book is the result of his many years of research and observation. In spite of his busy schedule, he has written this to bring benefit to others. It makes me very happy to see this book come out and I offer my sincerest good wishes that *MRCP II (Internal Medicine) Made Easy* will bring a tremendous amount of insight, knowledge and advancement for people in this field.

Tsem Tulku Rinpoche

INTRODUCTION

The theory part of the MRCP II is a difficult examination which separates the better from the good candidates, but overall a fair one. This book is designed for the changes in 1999 when multiple choice questions were introduced.

As the Associate College Tutor for the Royal College of Physicians of London and Instructor for the American Boards of Internal Medicine, I have always taught the candidates to think of the answer before looking at the choices. This appears counter-intuitive, but it allows the activation of the subconscious which is much faster than conscious cognition and enables the entire pattern to be understood intuitively as a Gestalt, thus experiencing the Eureka effect.

This is the expert method used in bedside clinical problem-solving by master clinicians and this book teaches this method. As you work through the book, you will subliminally learn this technique as one learns a melody. The basis of this approach is based on FMRI data and we are still in the infancy of the neuroscience revolution. This edge is critical as only 25-30% of candidates for the day will pass.

As I studied the literature of neuroscience, I was fascinated by a discussion wherein the late Carl Sagan asserted that all the features of evolution are beneficial and the Dalai Lama replied, "What about death?" These profound words made me realise the truism that humans are mortal as our genes are designed to have telomeres which do not regenerate and can only repair for a limited lifespan.

As I explored the source of the Dalai Lama's training and belief system, I realised that Buddha was one of the first Physicians as he used a "modern" medical approach which is to make: 1. the diagnosis (the fact that life is characterised by suffering), 2. the aetiology (based on our nature of clinging, pride, stupor and ignorance), 3. the prognosis (which is good), and 4. the treatment (the fact that there is a way out, the details of which are beyond the scope of this book). Although these words come from a source 2,500 years ago, it is as true today for all the candidates taking this exam, and the way out (in this particular context) is to master this book and the methodology therein.

As a Cardiologist and Physician who has searched for excellence in Medicine, I believe that Hippocrates spoke true when he said that "the

Art is long, but life is short" and all the modern temples of Medicine such as MGH (Harvard), that Dr. Samuel Shem called the "House of God," are merely preventing the inevitable.

For this reason, I have been fortunate to have come across the words of Buddha (Dharma) and found a teacher, who has been kinder than all my past dedicated Professors of Medicine as he has begun to teach me the Art and Science of how to achieve Ultimate happiness, which is the ultimate cure for the protean ailments of human existence. As it is said in the Yongen Shigurma, "The source of all inspiration is one's teacher." This book is no exception. I dedicate and offer this manuscript from an unworthy student to a kind and great teacher, His Eminence Tsem Tulku Rinpoche of Kechara House, Kuala Lumpur, Tsem Kacho Ling Malaysia and Gaden Shartse University, India.

As a brother Physician, I wish you the best of luck in your examinations, and a successful career.

Dr Chong Wei Min MRCP (U.K.) Cardiology Fellow (Harvard)
Consultant Interventional Cardiologist and Physician
Columbia Asia Hospital, Perak, Malaysia 2009

QUESTIONS & ANSWERS

Q 001

A 24-year-old university student is found unconscious. Next to him is a letter from the Royal College of Surgeons informing him that he has not passed his examinations. He appears clinically dehydrated and is hyperventilating.

Investigations showed:
- pH – 7.1
- Pa CO_2 – 1.3 kPa
- Pa O_2 – 1.7 kPa
- Urea – 12 mmols/L
- Glucose – 3 mmols/L
- Urinary ferric chloride (for reducing sugars) – red purple discolouration.

A. WHAT IS THE DIAGNOSIS?
ANS: This patient has metabolic acidosis due to salicylate intoxication. Serum salicylate levels and urinary pH estimation should be performed.

B. WHAT IS THE TREATMENT FOR THIS PATIENT?
ANS: The patient should undergo forced alkaline diuresis to bring the urinary pH to 8.

Q 002

A 54-year-old man undergoes an oral 75 g glucose tolerance test as part of the investigation for weight loss. He is having tremors and has visible goitre.

TIME (MINS)	BLOOD GLUCOSE (MMOLS/L)
0	4.8
30	13
45	7.4
60	4.6
90	3.4
120	4.1

A. WHAT IS THE DIAGNOSIS?

ANS: This patient has lag storage glucose tolerance test.

B. WHAT OTHER CONDITIONS MAY CAUSE A SIMILAR RESULT?

ANS: Gastrectomy, normal variant, severe liver disease and pregnancy.

Q 003

A 25-year-old Englishwoman in Egypt is admitted to a local hospital following a convulsion. Six weeks ago she gave birth to her first child and was diagnosed by the attending physician to be suffering from postnatal depression due to her inability to sleep. She was prescribed hypnotics and diazepam for daytime sedation. Several days after starting the therapy, she began to appear confused and complained of severe central abdominal pain. A day prior to the admission, she felt lightheaded and collapsed while visiting the pyramids of Giza; the following day she has a *grand mal* seizure and is admitted.

On examination, she is drowsy with evidence of mild left-sided weakness. She is pyrexial at 38°C, pulse at 120/min and BP at 180/120 mmHg. There is no visceromegaly, but the abdomen is tender. Pelvic examination is normal. She is unable to dorsiflex the left wrist and has a left foot drop. She complains of double vision on lateral gaze. Fundal examination is normal.

Initial investigation showed:
- Hb – 12 g/dl
- WBC – 14.8 x 10^9/L (70% neutrophils)
- Platelets – 315 x10^9/L
- Sodium – 136 mmols/L
- Potassium – 4.8 mmols/L
- Urea – 7.6 mmols/L
- Creatinine – 111 μmols/L
- Glucose – 5.2 mmols/L

A. WHAT IS THE DIAGNOSIS?

ANS: This patient has acute intermittent porphyria. Urine should be examined for porphobilinogen.

B. How would you treat this patient?

Ans: During acute attacks, narcotic analgesics may be required for abdominal pain and phenothiazines are useful for nausea, vomiting, anxiety and restlessness. Chlorhydrate can be given safely for insomnia. Benzodiazepines in low doses are probably safe if a minor tranquilliser is required. Intravenous heme is more effective than glucose in reducing porphyrin precursor excretion and leads to rapid recovery. The response to heme therapy is reduced if the initiation of this therapy is delayed. Heme arginate and heme albumin are chemically more stable than hematin and are less likely to produce inflammation of the veins or any anticoagulant effects.

The rate of recovery from an acute attack depends upon the degree of neuronal damage and may be rapid (1–2 days). Recovery from severe motor neuropathy may continue for months or years. Identification or avoidance of inciting factors can hasten recovery from an attack and prevent future attacks. Multiple inciting factors can contribute to a symptomatic episode. Frequent clear-cut cyclical attacks occur in some women and can be prevented with luteinising hormone releasing hormone analogue.

Q 004

A 45-year-old paediatrician is brought in unconscious to the accident and emergency department. He has had a previous episode of loss of consciousness and had become aggressive and irrational prior to the episode of loss of consciousness. He had been seen by his neighbour to have smashed car windows in the neighbourhood. His wife had left him because of his unstable personality. Since then he has become increasingly irrational and irritable. He eats plenty of sweets and snacks during the day in order to give up smoking; he has put on 20 kg since then. He has a history of lithotripsy for a kidney stone. He has four children who are all doing well. His father died at the age of 38 of a perforated peptic ulcer. His mother is well.

On examination, he is unarousable, with flaccid limbs. His reflexes are normal. His pupils are dilated but respond to light. The pulse is 120/min, regular; BP 150/90 mmHg; JVP normal and heart sounds are normal. Respiratory examination reveals some crackles in the right side of the chest and abdominal examination is normal.

A. WHAT IS THE IMMEDIATE MANAGEMENT OF THIS PATIENT?

ANS: One should treat the patient with 50–60% of dextrose intravenously and start antibiotics for presumed aspiration pneumonia.

B. WHAT IS THE DIAGNOSIS?

ANS: This patient has the MEN I syndrome and many of his symptoms are suggestive of insulinoma. This is also called Wermer's Syndrome.

It is the neoplastic transformation of parathyroid, pituitary and pancreatic islet cells. The syndrome is inherited as an autosomal dominant trait; therefore each child born to an affected parent has a 50% chance of inheriting the predisposing gene. Insulin secreting tumours may be localised by MRI or CT scan. Transhepatic venous catheterisation sample for insulin in the portal circulation may allow localisation of the tumour. Intra-operative ultrasound may also be used to localise these tumours.

C. WHAT FURTHER TESTS SHOULD BE PERFORMED?

ANS: One should perform a calcium level test to screen for an elevated PTH level, prolactin level as an intra-cerebral tumour pressing on the stalk may reduce dopamine (which is the inhibitor of prolactin release). The pressure on the stalk may increase the serum prolactin. One should also screen the children for calcium, prolactin and gut hormones.

D. WHAT CONDITION DID HIS FATHER DIE OF?

ANS: His father probably died of the Zollinger-Ellison Syndrome (gastrinoma). The ulcer diathesis is frequently refractory to conservative therapy such as antacids. The diagnosis of Zollinger-Ellison is made by the presence of increased acid secretion, an elevation of the basal gastrin secretion (generally greater than 1,000 pg/ml) or an exaggerated stimulatory response to either secretin or calcium. In the diagnosis of the Z-E syndrome, other causes of elevated serum calcium such as achlorhydria, treatment with an H2-receptor antagonist, therapy with omeprazole, retained gastric antrum, small bowel re-section, gastric outlet obstruction and hypercalcemia should be excluded.

One third of patients with pancreatic islet cell tumours have insulin overproduction resulting in hypoglycaemia. This may cause bizarre behaviour, excessive hunger, weight gain, seizures and loss of consciousness in the fasting state. The diagnosis can be established by the documentation of hypoglycaemia during a short fast with simultaneous inappropriate elevation of insulin and C-peptide concentration.

E. What is the most common manifestation of this condition?
Ans: Hyperparathyroidism is the most common manifestation of the MEN I syndrome. Hypercalcemia may be detected during the teenage years and by the age of 40 most carriers are likely to be affected. Screening for hyperparathyroidism is enhanced by measurement of either an albumin adjusted or ionised serum calcium. The diagnosis is established by the finding of elevated serum calcium and intact parathyroid hormone levels. The clinical features of hyperparathyroidism in patients with MEN I do not differ substantially from those suffering from sporadic hyperparathyroidism and may include calcium containing kidney stones, bone abnormalities, gastro-intestinal and musculo-skeletal complaints.

F. One of the patient's children has uncontrollable diarrhoea and occasional irregular heart beats. What is the most likely cause of this?
Ans: He probably has the Werner Morrison Syndrome. This is also known as the watery diarrhoea syndrome. It comprises watery diarrhoea, hyperkalemia (which causes the dysrrhythmia), hypochlohydria and systemic acidosis. The diarrhoea can be voluminous and is associated with an islet cell tumour; thereby the term 'pancreatic cholera' is often used although the syndrome is not restricted to pancreatic islet tumours and has been observed in association with carcinoid or other tumours.

There is considerable evidence that this tumour is caused by overproduction of VIP although the plasma concentration of this peptide may rarely be normal. Hypercalcemia is common and is thought to be the effect of VIP on bone.

Q 005

A 45-year-old swimming instructor is referred with poorly controlled hypertension. She also complains of malaise and tiredness. She has been on hypertensive therapy for 15 years and has been treated with multiple drugs to control her blood pressure but this was never achieved because of poor compliance. Recently the patient had fallen into the pool and complained of several episodes of giddiness brought on by exertion.

There is no history of palpitations, exertional dyspnoea or angina. Her husband complains she keeps him awake with her nocturia and headache that she has had for several years.

On examination, she is overweight, pulse is 75/min in sinus rhythm, BP is 222/122 mmHg supine and 160/90 mmHg on standing. The JVP is not raised and the apex is thrusting in quality. Auscultation reveals an ejection systolic murmur best heard at the apex without radiation. The chest is clear to auscultation. A one cm liver edge is palpable in the abdomen. Fundal examination reveals arterio-venous nipping, but the rest of the physical examination does not reveal any other abnormalities.

Initial investigations showed:
- Hb – 12 g/dl
- WBC – 7 x 10⁹/L
- Platelets – 450 x 10⁹/L
- Sodium – 144 mmols/L
- Potassium – 2.8 mmols/L
- Urea – 9.6 mmols/L
- Creatinine – 146 µmols/L
- Glucose – 4.3 mmols/L
- Spot urinary sodium – 27 mmols/L
- Spot urinary potassium – 48 mmols/L
- Urinary pH – neutral to alkaline (due to excessive secretion of ammonium and bicarbonate ions)
- Chest X-ray shows a moderately enlarged heart with a prominent left ventricular border. ECG shows sinus rhythm with evidence of left ventricular hypertrophy and a strain pattern.

A. WHAT IS THE DIAGNOSIS?

ANS: The most likely diagnosis is Conn's syndrome (primary hyperaldosteronism). One should also rule out idiopathic hyperplasia (bilateral) and essential hypertension over-treated with diuretics.

The patient should be treated with a 24-hour urinary aldosterone estimation, the lying and standing renin and aldosterone levels. The aldosterone level falls on standing in an adenoma but rises on standing in hyperplasia. One should then perform either a CT scan or an MRI to look for suprarenal adenoma. In a majority of cases, it is usually a unilateral adenoma, usually small and occurring with equal frequency on either side. The ECG and CXR evidence of left ventricular hypertrophy is secondary to the hypertension.

The criteria for the diagnosis of Conn's syndrome are:
i)   Diastolic hypertension without oedema
ii) Hyposecretion of renin (as judged by a low plasma renin activity level) that fails to increase appropriately during depletion (upright posture, sodium depletion)
iii) Hypersecretion of aldosterone that fails to suppress appropriately during volume expansion (such as during salt loading)

Patients with primary hyperaldosteronism do not have oedema since they exhibit an aldosterone escape phenomenon from the sodium retaining aspect of the minerocorticosteroids. If there is pretibial oedema, one should consider the possibilities of nephropathy and azotemia. The failure of plasma renin activity to rise normally during a volume depletion manoeuvre is criteria for primary aldosteronism; suppressed renin activity also occurs in about 25% of patients with essential hypertension. Once hyposecretion of renin and failure to suppress aldosterone are demonstrated, localisation of aldosterone secreting adenomas may be determined pre-operatively by a CT scan or by a percutaneous, transfemoral bilateral adrenal vein catheterisation with simultaneous adrenal venography. The latter technique permits radiologic localisation. In addition the adrenal vein may sometimes demonstrate a 2–3 fold rise in plasma aldosterone concentration on the involved side compared with the uninvolved side.

In cases of hyperaldosteronism secondary to cortical nodular hyperplasia, no localisation is found. It is vital for samples to be obtained at the time if possible and for cortisol levels to be measured to ensure that false localisation do not reflect an ACTH or stress induced rise in the aldosterone level.

B. How will you treat this patient?
Ans: Primary hyperaldosteronism due to adenoma is treated by surgical extirpation. Dietary sodium restriction and the administration of an aldosterone antagonist such as spironolactone may be effective.

Hypertension and hyperkalaemia are usually controlled by 25–100 mg spironolactone eight hourly. Patients have been managed successfully for years, but chronic therapy in man is limited by the development of breasts enlargement, decreased libido and impotence.

When idiopathic bilateral hyperplasia is suspected, surgery is indicated only when significant symptomatic hyperkalaemia cannot be controlled with medical therapy, for example, by spironolactone, triamterene or amiloride; hypertension associated with idiopathic hyperplasia is usually not benefited by bilateral adrenolectomy.

Q 006

A 30-year-old Indonesian lady is referred by a general practitioner. She complains of increased tiredness since being separated from her husband three years previously. She often feels tired and dizzy. She finds it increasingly difficult to bring up her three toddlers. She believes her husband left her for a much younger woman because her skin had become darker. Her periods have become irregular and her skin has become more pigmented. Her father was an insulin-dependant diabetic. She does not smoke or drink alcohol.

Examination reveals buccal pigmentation. The pulse is 60 beats/min and regular. Blood pressure 90/40 mmHg lying and 74 mmHg systolic when standing. The remainder of the examinations does not reveal any other findings.

The initial investigations:
- Hb – 9.6 g/dl
- MCV – 8.4 fl
- WBC – 4.6 x 10^9/L
- Platelet – 310 x 10^9/L
- Sodium – 130 mmol/L
- Potassium – 5.8 mmol/L
- Urea – 5.6 mmol/L
- Creatinine – 90 µmols/L
- Glucose – 4 mmol/L

A. WHAT IS THE DIAGNOSIS?
ANS: Polyendocrinopathy type II

Type I diabetes mellitus is the most common manifestation of polyglandular autoimmune syndrome type II. It occurs in approximately 50% of affected families. Mucocutaneous candidiasis does not occur. This condition tends to develop later in life and was first described by Schmidt in patients who have lymphocytic infiltration of the adrenal and thyroid glands at autopsy and who have family members with type I diabetes and hypogonadism.

The buccal pigmentation and the electrolyte changes are highly suggestive of Addison's disease. The hypothyroidism may account for the anaemia. The auto-immune thyroid disease causes either Hashimoto's thyroiditis or hypothyroidism. However, many patients with anti-microsomal and anti-thyroglobulin antibodies never develop abnormalities of thyroid function. Thus, these antibodies alone are poor predictors of future disease. Dermatological manifestations include vitiligo, alopecia totalis and alopecia areata. Antibodies against the melanocytes may explain localised areas of de-pigmentation. A few patients may develop transient hypoparathyroidism with hypercalcaemia as a result of antibodies that block the action of parathyroid hormone.

Up to a quarter of patients may present with myasthenia gravis and an even higher percentage present with myasthenia with a thymoma and thus have polyglandular autoimmune syndrome type II.

B. WHAT FURTHER INVESTIGATIONS SHOULD BE PERFORMED?
ANS: One should perform:
i) A Synacthen test
ii) T_3, T_4, TSH
iii) Cortisol level
iv) X-ray of the abdomen for calcification of the adrenals or an MRI of the abdomen.

Q 007

A 43-year-old manager of a pharmacy, who had an uncomplicated appendicectomy, collapsed in the ward on the 4th post-operative day after feeling dizzy. Her vital signs were stable at the time. Pulse was 70/min, regular, BP 90/60 mmHg. The house officer checked her blood glucose and found it to be 2.3 mmols/L. She was treated with IV dextrose after which she felt better. Since that time she requires continuous infusion of glucose to stop her from being hypoglycaemic. She mentions she has felt dizzy since the operation and that she often felt dizzy following micturation even before her operation. She had collapsed once while micturating. Her history includes a cholecystectomy at the age of 20, an emergency caesarean section for placenta previa following her 4th pregnancy and premature menopause at the age of 35. She was unable to lactate after the emergency caesarean section and the child had to be bottle-fed. She gave no relevant family history. She is married with four children, age 15, 11, 10 and six, with an adopted Tibetan boy. Her husband works as a detective in the local police department. She smokes 15 cigarettes daily and drinks alcohol socially.

Examination reveals a pale woman with bradycardia, a pulse rate of 50/min, a blood pressure of 90/70 mmHg with no postural drop. The JVP is raised, heart sounds are normal. Respiratory and abdominal examination does not reveal any abnormalities. The axillary and pubic hair is absent and she denies either shaving or plucking the hairs.

The pre-operative investigations reveal:
- WBC – 4.5 x 10^9/L
- Platelet – 210x 10^9/L
- Sodium – 130 mmol/L
- Potassium – 5.8 mmol/L
- Urea – 4.8 mmol/L
- Creatinine – 82 µmols/L

A. WHAT IS THE LIKELY DIAGNOSIS?
ANS: Sheehan's syndrome (Post-partum pituitary necrosis)

Patients with diabetes mellitus are susceptible to peripartum infarction even in the absence of significant haemorrhage. Post-partum pituitary infarction occurs in the setting of haemorrhage with systemic hypotension. The enlarged pituitary gland during pregnancy may be more vulnerable to ischaemia.

The condition is sometimes diagnosed years after the event, but the inability to lactate is the most important initial clue. Clinical diabetes insipidus is rare in this setting. Auto-immune pituitary destruction may also occur during late pregnancy, but it is often associated with elevated prolactin level. The lateral wing of the pituitary has a precarious blood-supply; most lactotropes reside in this area. This explains why failure of lactation is often the earliest clue to panhypopituitarism, resulting from pituitary infarction during the peripartum period. Diabetes insipidus may appear during pregnancy and cease a few days after delivery or it may commence after parturition in women with Sheehan's syndrome and there is a relationship with cortisol deficiency.

Q 008

A 57-year-old physician has difficulty in climbing stairs. His medical history is unremarkable. On systemic inquiry, he admits to an early morning smoker's cough.

On examination, he is overweight and BP is 150/90 mmHg and he has evidence of symmetrical weakness of hip flexion. All reflexes are present and there is no sensory abnormality. The serum cortisol measurement at 9 am is 916 nanomols/L, at midnight 886 nanomols/L. After 2 milligrams of dexamethasone 6-hourly for 48 hours, the 9 am serum cortisol is 786 nanomols/L.

A. WHAT IS THE DIFFERENTIAL DIAGNOSIS?
ANS: It is Cushing's syndrome due to ectopic ACTH or due to an adrenal tumour.

Q 009

A 25 month old boy is being investigated for recurrent attacks of acute otitis media and chest infections.

- Hb – 13 g/dl
- WBC – 6 x 10⁹/L (78% neutrophils, 27% lymphocytes)
- Platelets – 360 x 10⁹/l
- Albumin – 37 g/L
- IgG – 10 g/L
- IgM – 1.5 g/L

A. GIVE TWO POSSIBLE DIAGNOSES TO ACCOUNT FOR THE RECURRENT INFECTIONS.
ANS: This patient either has selective IgA deficiency which may be associated with bronchiectasis or cystic fibrosis.

The tenacious secretion in the bronchi is associated with impaired clearance resulting in colonisation and recurrent infection with a variety of organisms, particularly mucoid strains of Pseudomonas aeruginosa. Other organisms include staphylococcus aureus, haemophilus influenza, E. coli and P. cepacia. Additional respiratory tract complications in cystic fibrosis include recurrent pneumo phoresis, sinusitis and nasal polyps. Males are generally infertile due to atresia of the vas deferens.

B. What two investigations should be performed?
Ans: Measurement of the serum IgA level and the serum sweat test.

IgA deficiency in association with ciliary dysfunction is termed as primary ciliary dyskinesia. In selective IgA deficiency, the patient may have Kartagener's syndrome in which *situs inversus* accompanies bronchiectasis and sinusitis. It has been hypothesised that ciliary motility is necessary for the proper rotation of the viscera during embryogenesis so that viscero-rotation is random when normal ciliary function is lost.

Between 1–2% of patients with the clinical syndrome of cystic fibrosis have normal sweat chloride levels. In most of these patients, the nasal transepithelial potential difference (PD) is raised into the diagnostic range of cystic fibrosis as sweat acini do not secrete in response to injected beta adrenergic agonist. The diagnosis of cystic fibrosis rests on the combination of clinical criteria and the analysis of sweat chloride levels. The value of the sodium and chloride concentration in sweat may vary with age, but in adults chloride concentration of more than 70 milliequivalent/L, discriminates between cystic fibrosis patients and other patients with similar lung disease.

Q 010

A 35-year-old man with a 6-year history of insulin-dependant diabetes is noted to have the following results:
- Resting heart rate – 96/min, heart rate variation with deep inspiration 4 breaths/min (normally more than 15/min)
- Valsalva ratio – 1:1

A. What is the significance of these results?
Ans: It suggests the patient has autonomic neuropathy.

Q 011

A routine 75 g glucose tolerance test of pre-university students yields the following results:

Time (min)	Plasma (mmols/L)
0	-7.8
120	-10.6

A. What is the diagnosis?
Ans: It implies an impaired glucose tolerance test.

B. What percentage of these patients, if followed for 10 years, will develop diabetes?
Ans: 2.4%/year will develop diabetes.

Q 012

A 43-year-old schizophrenic man is admitted for investigation of painless jaundice.

- Investigation results:
- Sodium – 129 mmol/L
- Potassium – 4 mmol/L
- Urea – 4.2 mmol/L
- Bilirubin – 76 micromol/L
- AST – 60 IU/L
- Alkaline phosphatase – 656 IU/L
- Albumin – 40 g/L
- Plasma protein – 54 g/L
- Hb – 12 g/dl
- WBC – 11 x 10^9/L (60% neutrophil, 24% lymphocytes)
- Platelets – 253 x 10^9/L

A. What is the diagnosis?
Ans: Phenothiazine induced cholestatic jaundice.

In about 1% of patients receiving chlorpromazine, intrahepatic cholestasis with jaundice develops about 1–4 weeks after therapy. There are instances where jaundice occurs after a single exposure. Pruritis may preceed the appearance of jaundice, dark urine and light stools.

Eosinophilia with or without mild leucocytosis may be present, and conjugated hyperbilirubinaemia, a moderately elevated serum alkaline phosphatase level and a mild elevation of the serum amino transferase level (100–200 units) may be noted.

Liver biopsy reveals cholestasis, bile plaques in bile canaliculi and dense infiltrates of polymorphonuclear, eosinophilic and mononuclear leucocytes. Occasionally, scattered foci of hepatic parenchymal necrosis may be evident. Jaundice and pruritis usually subsides within 4–8 weeks following cessation of therapy, and are usually without sequelae, and fatalities are rare. Cholestyramine may be of value in relieving severe pruritis. In a small number of patients, jaundice is prolonged for several months to years; a disorder resembling, but distinct from, primary biliary cirrhosis may develop, but it is rare.

B. THIS PATIENT UNDERGOES SURGERY FOR RUPTURED AORTIC ANEURYSM A YEAR LATER, COMPLICATED BY HYPOTENSION AND HYPOXAEMIA. HE DEVELOPS JAUNDICE ON THE 2ND POST-OPERATIVE DAY. THE SERUM BILIRUBIN IS PREDOMINANTLY CONJUGATED AND IS 350 MICROMOL/L. BY THE 8TH DAY, THE SERUM ALKALINE PHOSPHATASE IS ELEVATED 3-FOLD. THE PATIENT'S AST AND SGOT ARE ONLY MILDLY ELEVATED. WHAT IS THE DIAGNOSIS?

ANS: Benign post-operative intrahepatic cholestasis. The pathophysiology of this form of post-operative cholestatic jaundice is uncertain. The liver morphlogy is striking in that necrosis is not seen, only cholestasis and erythrophagocytosis.

However, it probably reflects:
i)   Increased pigment load.
ii) Decreased liver function due to hypoxaemia and hypotension
iii) Decreased renal bilirubin excretion due to varying degrees of tabular necrosis as a result of shock.

The diagnostic possibility must be considered in post-operative patients with marked cholestatic jaundice. The course of the jaundice is self-limiting and will subside if the other systemic complications do not predominate and lead to death.

C. THE LUNG SPIROMETRY SHOWS THE FOLLOWING DATA:
FEVI – 3 LIT (6 LITRES)
FVC – 3.2 LIT (5.8 LITRES)

WHAT IS THE RESPIRATORY DEFECT?
ANS: This is a restrictive lung defect.

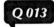

A 55-year salt miner who presented with oliguria three hours after a cross clamping and Dacron repair of an abdominal aortic aneurysm at the hospital.

The serum electrolytes:
- Sodium – 144 ummol/L
- Urea – 14.5 mmol/l
- Creatinine – 130 μmol/L
- Potassium – 4.0 mmol/L
- Urinary osmolality of 600 mOsm/kg

A. WHAT IS THE DIAGNOSIS?
ANS: It is pre-renal azotemia.

This definitive diagnosis of pre-renal azotemia can only be made when renal perfusion results in poor resolution of acute renal failure. Typically, the urine sodium is less than 5 mmol/L, a concentration supported by the demonstration of avid urinary sodium retention by the kidney. The urinary sediment is unremarkable.

Potassium is usually not required unless sodium bicarbonate is administered for moderate to severe acidosis. Cardiac failure may require aggressive management with anti-arrhythmic drug agents, pre-load and after-load reducing agents or mechanical aids such as intra-aortic balloon therapy to augment cardiovascular function; intravascular coronary perfusion may be improved.

Q 014

A 45-year-old man is referred with pain in his leg and difficulty in climbing stairs. He has recently been sacked and is separated from his wife. He smokes 20 cigarettes a day and drinks alcohol in large volume. He socialises frequently with his clients and is on omeprazole for peptic ulcer. He has had a cough for the last two months and he coughed out some blood a few weeks ago. He is not taking medication.

On examination, the patient is plethoric and thin. Early Dupuytren's contracture is noted on the left hand. Cardiovascular examination is normal. His abdomen is soft and there is no visible organomegaly. Wasting of leg muscles is noted. His knee and ankle jerks are absent and pin-prick sensation finished below the knees.

Investigations showed:
- Hb – 13.9 g/dl
- MCV – 109 f1
- WBC – 5 x 10⁹/L
- Ptatelet – 180 x 10⁹/L
- Sodium – 138 mmmol/l
- Potassium – 5 mmol/l
- Urea – 5 mmol/L
- Bilirubin – 16 μmol/l
- AST – 50 IU/L
- Gamma glutamyl – 90 IU/L
- Alkaline phosphatase – 80 IU/L
- Glucose – 4 mmol/L
- Creatinine phosphokinase – 45 IU/L
- Chest X-ray is normal

A. LIST TWO POSSIBLE CAUSES OF THE PATIENT'S SIGNS.
ANS: Alcoholism and malignancy.

B. WHAT IS THE MOST LIKELY DIAGNOSIS?
ANS: Alcoholic neuropathy and myopathy.

A chronic alcoholic may develop painful myopathy with myoglobinuria after a bout of heavy drinking, or may present a painless acute hyperkalaemic myopathy which is completely reversible, or may show an asymptomatic elevation serum CK and myoglobin. Acute muscle weakness with myoglobinuria may occur in prolonged severe hypokalaemia, due to patossium loss or hypophosphataemia and hypomagnesemia often seen in chronic alchoholics and in patients on nasogastric suction receiving parenteral hyperalimentation. An acute necrotising myopathy with myoglobinuria may accompany hypernatraemia.

Q 015

WHAT IS THE HOLIDAY HEART SYNDROME?

ANS: This is a condition, with atrial fibrillation, which typically appears after binge drinking. It is frequently followed by atrial flutter and ventricular premature depolarisation. Other patients may develop left ventricular hypertrophy related to systemic hypertension. They may present symptoms of pulmonary congestion due to abnormal diastolic stiffness (diminished compliance of the left ventricle)

This must be differentiated from alcoholic cardiomyopathy. An individual who consumes a large quantity of alcohol over the years may develop a clinical picture identical to idiopathic dilated cardiomyopathy. Abstinence from alcohol before heart failure develops may halt the progression or even reverse the course of the disease, unlike the idiopathic variety, which is marked by progressive deterioration. Alcoholics with advance heart failure have a poor prognosis, especially if they continue to drink. Less than one quarter survive three years.

The key to treatment of alcoholic cardiomyopathy is total and permanent abstinence. Although thiamine deficiency may be present in some of these patients, alcoholic cardiomyopathy is associated with a low cardiac output and systemic vasoconstriction. In contrast, Beri-beri heart disease does not appear to cause alcoholic cardiomyopathy. The toxic effect of alcohol on striated muscle often extends beyond the heart to cause myopathy in the skeletal muscles.

Q 016

A 48-year-old lady had an MI four years ago and underwent a successful coronary bypass grafting. Bilateral arcus senilis was noted during surgery and the fasting lipids showed elevated cholesterol. She smokes 30 cigarettes a day and drinks one glass of brandy every night. She noticed the skin on her chest was becoming thicker and she had symptoms suggestive of Raynaud's syndrome.

Examination reveals a pulse of 110 beats/min and blood pressure of 120/80 mmHg lying and 110/60 mmHg sitting. There is mild ulnar deviation of the fingers and the SHO noted she has clubbing. Auscultation of lung bases reveal bibasal crackles, but she does not complain of much sputum production. Abdominal examination reveals a smoothly enlarged liver; there is epigastric discomfort and rectal examination reveals smooth brown stools.

- Hb – 11 g/d1
- WBC – 16 x 10⁹/L
- Ptatelet – 240 x 10⁹/L
- Sodium – 135 mmols/L
- Potassium – 5 mmomls/L
- Urea – 9 mmols/L
- Creatinine – 110 µmols/L
- PT – 15 sec
- PTTK – 33 sec
- Bilirubin – 30 µmols/L
- Aspartate tranaminase – 76 IU/L
- Alkaline phosphatase – 1,350 IU/L
- Gamma glutamyl transferase – 1,120 IU/L
- Albumin – 32 g/L
- Total protein – 80 g/L
- Calcium – 2.2 mmols/L
- Phosphate – 0.9 mmols/L

A. WHAT IS THE DIAGNOSIS?

ANS: This patient has a combination of primary biliary cirrhosis, and scleroderma, associated with fibrosing alveolitis, portal hypertension (with oesophageal varices), acid peptic disease, Raynaud's disease, hyperlipideamia and coronary artery disease.

B. HOW WILL YOU DIAGNOSE THE HEPATIC CONDITION?

ANS: This should be considered in a middle-aged woman with unexplained pruritus or elevated alkaline phosphatase and presenting with a clinical or laboratory picture of impairment of biliary excretion. A positive serum anti-mitochondrial antibody determination provides important diagnostic evidence. False positive results occur; therefore a liver biopsy must be performed to confirm the diagnosis.

The biliary tract should be evaluated to exclude remediable extrahepatic biliary tract obstruction, especially in view of the frequent presence of co-existing cholelithiasis. The liver biopsy will show chronic non-suppurative destructive cholangitis. This is a necrotising inflammation of the portal triad. It is characterised by the destruction of the medium and small bile ducts, a dense infiltrate of acute and chronic inflammatory cells, mild fibrosis and occasional bile stasis. At times, periductal granulomas and lymph follicles are found adjacent to bile ducts.

Subsequently, the inflammatory infiltrate becomes less prominent, the number of bile duct is reduced and smaller bile ductules proliferate (stage II). Progression over months and years lead to decreased interlobular ducts, loss of liver cells and expansion of periportal fibrosis into a network of connective scar-tissue (stage III). Ultimately, cirrhosis, which may be micronodular or macronodular, develops. This is the terminal stage (stage IV).

Q 017

A 46-year-old woman who teaches English and Spanish is admitted comatose. The history taken from her long-time companion reveals she was diagnosed as non-insulin dependant diabetic eight years ago and suffers from arthritis. She does not smoke and drinks sherry with her evening meals. Her conscious level had deteriorated over the last week.

On examination she appears sun-tanned (the companion says she is a writer and usually stays indoors). She is responsive to pain with an extensor plantar response and there are symmetrical brisk reflexes. There is normal blood pressure.

- Glucose – 5 mmols/L
- Sodium – 126 mmols/L
- Potassium – 2.9 mmol/L
- Urea – 1.8 mmol/L
- CSF
  · protein – 0.6 g/L
  · glucose – 4 mmol/L
  · cell-count – 5/cubic mm

A. WHAT IS THE LIKELY CAUSE OF HER COMA?

ANS: The colour change of the skin is due to increased iron or bronze discolouration resulting from melanin deposition in haemochromatosis.

Slight deterioration of the intellect and minimal personality change suggest hepatocellular disease or the presence of porto-systemic venous shunt, but care must be taken to exclude other causes such as neurological diseases.

The presence of flapping tremors of the hands may be found in porto-systemic encephalopathy or impending hepatic coma.

B. WHAT INVESTIGATIONS WOULD YOU PERFORM?
Ans: Iron studies, liver biopsy, serum ammonia level, EEG.

C. HOW WOULD YOU MANAGE THIS PATIENT?
ANS: I would rule out any reversible causes and start the patient on a combination of lactulose and neomycin.

The patient should be put on a glucose infusion to prevent hypoglycaemia and the rest of the management depends on the course of the patient's condition. One should treat haemochromatosis with venesection.

D. HOW WOULD YOU TREAT THE PRIMARY DISORDER?
ANS: Genetic haemochromatosis involves the removal of excess body iron and supportive treatment of damaged organs. Iron is best removed by twice weekly phlebotomy of 500 ml. The plasma transferrin level remains high until the available iron stores are depleted. In contrast, the plasma ferritin concentration falls progressively, reflecting the gradual decrease in body iron stores. When the transferrin saturation and the ferritin levels become normal, phlebotomies are performed to maintain the level at a normal range. The measures become abnormal with iron re-accumulation.

Chelating agents such as desferroxamine, when given parenterally, remove 10–20 mg of iron/day. Phlebotomy is also less expensive, more convenient and safer for most patients. Chelating agents are indicated when anaemia or hypoprotinaemia is severe enough to preclude phlebotomy. Subcutaneous infusion of desferrioxamine using a portable pump is the most effective means of administration. The management of hepatic failure, heart failure and diabetes mellitus differs little from the conventional management of these conditions. Loss of libido and change of secondary sexual characteristics are partially relieved by parenteral administration of testosterone or gonadotropin.

Q 018

A 43-year-old Turkish lady is sent to Casualty by her practitioner because of persistent fever, the cause of which could not be determined despite multiple investigations. Four months ago she had married a gentleman while attending a conference in India. During the conference, she had felt unwell and had evening rise of temperature which has been persistent since her return. She has lost 2 kg in weight, feels lethargic, weak and comments that there is an increased effort for her to climb to her penthouse apartment at night (the lifts have not been working since last week). Two weeks prior to admission, she had a sharp pain on the left side of the abdomen which had settled with opiates which required observation overnight in hospital. She has a history of pulmonary tuberculosis six years ago treated with therapy for six months. There was a left-sided deep vein thrombosis which was treated and she has a regular migraine.

On examination, she has a temperature of 38°C, pulse 110/min regular, blood pressure 150/90 mmHg. Splinter haemorrhages was noted on the left second finger and on the left 4th finger. Cardiovascular, respiratory, abdominal and neurological systems are normal.

Investigations:
- Hb – 8 g/dl
- MCV – 100 fl
- Platelet – 92 x 10⁹/L
- WBC – 3.8 x 10⁹/L (90% neutrophils)
- ESR – 100 mm in the 1st hour
- Sodium – 130 mmols/L
- Potassium – 5.2 mmols/L
- Urea – 8 mmol/L
- Creatinine – 113 µmols/L
- Glucose – 6 mmols/L
- AST – 92 IU/L
- Bilirubin – 22 µmols/L
- Alkaline phosphatase – 115 IU/L
- Corrected calcium – 2.24 mmol/L
- Phosphate – 0.9 mmol/L
- Chest X-ray – Right apical shadowing consistent with previous TB
- MSU – Blood + protein +++

A. What are the different diagnoses?
Ans: One should consider sub-acute bacterial endocarditis, reactivation of TB and SLE.

B. What is the most likely diagnosis?
Ans: SLE with splenic infarction

C. List three investigations you would perform to confirm your diagnosis.
Ans: Double stranded DNA, the complement level test and the anticardiolipin antibodies, anti-SM antibodies.

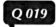

A 50-year-old woman, who had an elder brother who died of a subarachnoid haemorrhage, has the following blood count:

- Hb – 22 g/dl
- PVC – 70%
- MCV – 83 fl
- MCHC – 30 g/dl
- Platelets – 145 x 10⁹/L
- WBC – 9 x 10⁹/L

Other investigations:
- Urea and electrolytes are normal
- PO_2 – 11.1 kPa
- PCO_2 – 26 kPa

The ophthalmologist noted capillary angiomas that are causing a gradual deterioration of her vision. She is also unstable on her feet and it was thought she was drunk.

A. What is the likely diagnosis?
Ans: Polycythaemia secondary to ectopic erythropoietin production from a cerebellar haemangioblastoma.
Cerebellar haemangioblasma may occur in clusters and are slow-growing cystic tumours. This may also occur in the medulla or the spinal cord; enlargement of the cerebellar tumour may lead to obstructive

hydrocephalus with headache, papilloedema and cerebellar ataxia.

The tumour usually does not become symptomatic before adolescence, but the diagnosis must be considered in all adults with cerebellar tumour. An association with renal cell carcinoma led to the localisation of the mutant gene on chromosome 3. The mutant gene has been recently identified. The polycythaemia, as a result of ectopic production of erythropoietin by the haemangioblastoma, may disappear after the excision of the tumour.

B. WHAT ARE THE DIFFERENTIAL DIAGNOSES WHICH MAY CAUSE A SIMILAR HAEMOTOLOGICAL PROFILE?

ANS: One should consider a renal tumour, renal cyst, uterine fibroma and hepatomas.

Q 020

A 22-year-old cardiologist, complains of very severe pain in the finger joints, knees and ankles. This has been present for the last two weeks. He had fever two weeks ago, which lasted for one week. There is tenderness over the affected joints and muscle insertion, but no swelling. There is no pruritic maculopapular rash. He has returned to the United Kingdom having worked in South East Asia.

A. WHAT THREE INVESTIGATIONS WOULD YOU PERFORM?

ANS: Culture, thick and thin blood film.

B. WHAT THREE DIAGNOSES WOULD BE RESPONSIBLE?

ANS: Rickets, relapsing fever, dengue fever, malaria and meningococcal septicaemia.

Severe falciparum malaria is a medical emergency that requires intensive nursing care and expert management. One should contact the London School of Tropical Medicine and Hygiene. If the patients are comatose, their blood glucose levels should be checked and they should be positioned on their right side. The choice of drug dosage and the route of administration depends on the prevailing sensitivity of the plasmodium falciparum to antimalarial drügs, the condition of the patient and the place where the treatment is given. Quinine is the main treatment because of its action against chloroquine resistant strains of plasmodium falciparum.

Quinidine gluconate is as effective as quinine and is more readily available outside tropical areas. In the United States, quinidine has replaced quinine for the parenteral treatment of severe malaria. Quinidine is more cardiotoxic than quinine. Its administration must be closely monitored for dysrrhythmia and hypotension must be avoided. A blood level in excess of 22 µmmols/L, an electrocardiographic QT interval of more than 0.55 sec, a QRS prolongation of more than 50% or a QT of more than 25% of baseline, is an indication for slowing the infusion rate. One should remember that quinine can cause hypoglycaemia and this should be treated.

The kidney function should be accessed daily. The management of fluid balance is difficult in severe malaria because there is a thin line between overhydration, which can lead to pulmonary oedema, and underhydration, which can contribute to renal impairment. If necessary, pulmonary arterial wedge pressure may need to be monitored.(The use of the Swan Ganz has not been shown to reduce mortality in the ICU). The pressure should be maintained in the low to normal range. As soon as the patient can take fluids, oral antimalarials should be given.

The treatment of dengue fever is entirely symptomatic and in the absence of dengue haemorrhagic fever or dengue shock syndrome, there is no danger of mortality. Dengue haemorrhagic fever is common in Malaysia and the illness begins abruptly. Petechiae are most frequently located at the forehead and the distal extremities. It is critical to perform twice daily platelet counts, D-dimer test (or FDP), Beeding Time, Clotting Time and INR. Extremities are frequently cyanosed and there may be hypotension with narrowing of the pulse pressure and tachycardia. Most fatalities occurs in the 4th or 5th day of illness. There may be malaena, haematemesis, coma or unresponsive shock, all poor prognostic signs. Cyanosis, dyspnoea and convulsions are terminal manifestations.

After this critical period, survivors show steady and rapid improvement. Over 500 cases of dengue haemorrhagic fever have been reported with major epidemics in China, Vietnam, Indonesia, Malaysia, Thailand and Cuba. In the Cuban outbreak in 1981, almost 35,000 people developed dengue. Approximately 10,000 had haemorrhagic manifestation and 158 died. Studies in Thailand have estimated that the frequency of dengue shock syndrome is 11 cases per 1,000 secondary dengue infections. It occurs more often in girls than in boys. Dengue haemorrhagic fever occurs almost exclusively in indigenous populations. It has been observed only rarely in Whites or Europeans, despite the common occurance of classic dengue in this group. Dengue is also a problem in parts of America.

At present, vector control is the only measure available to control haemorrhagic fever. The author believes in early replacement of blood components in DHF with aggressive fluid therapy with a vigilance and readiness to treat fluid overload as there is a period of spontaneous leakiness of all the blood vessels of the body.

Q 021

The 60-year-old wife of a farmer is referred to the hospital because of lethargy, weight loss and pain. She complains of stiffness in her limb girdle.

On questioning, she complains she has pain in her knees, wrists and ankles and paraesthesia in her hands. She has a palpable lymph node in the neck.

A. WHAT TWO DIAGNOSES ARE LIKELY?
ANS: Myxoedema, polymyalgia rheumatica (with giant cell arteritis)

B. WHAT OTHER RADIOLOGICAL INVESTIGATIONS WOULD YOU PERFORM?
ANS: I would like to do a sketetal survey to look for chondrocalcinosis.

C. HOW WOULD YOU TREAT THIS PATIENT?
ANS: After assessing the thyroid function, one may need to treat the thyroid insufficiency and administer prednisolone.

D. WHAT THREE CLINICAL TESTS WOULD HELP YOU IN YOUR DIAGNOSIS?
ANS:
i) Assessment of the reflexes
ii) Feel for the temporal arteries, and if hardened, requires a biopsy. The pathology of this condition is patchy and a negative biopsy does not rule out the diagnosis.
iii) Lymph node biopsy (for the paraneoplastic syndrome).

Q 022

A 29-year-old Singaporean air-hostess has pain in her upper limbs and neck; this has spread to her knees and jaw. The joints and muscles are tender without swelling. She is regularly massaged by her male companion. She has noticed her fingers become pale in the cold weather in London and her eyes are painful. She is on no medication except the oral contraceptive pill. The general practitioner is able to take her blood pressure in her left arm.

A. WHAT THREE DIAGNOSES SHOULD BE CONSIDERED?
ANS: Mixed connective tissue disease, Takayasu's disease and polyarteritis nodosa.

B. HOW WOULD YOU INVESTIGATE HER?
ANS: An aortic arch aortogram, ESR, antibodies to the double stranded DNA, and P anca.

C. SEVERAL MONTHS LATER, IT WAS DISCOVERED SHE HAS A RARE FORM OF LEUKAEMIA. WHAT DIAGNOSIS WOULD YOU CONSIDER?
ANS: Hairy cell leukaemia can be associated with classical polyarteritis nodosa.

The pathogenic mechanism of this association is unclear. The presence of hepatitis B antigenaemia is in approximately 30% of patients with systemic vasculitis, particularly of the classic PAN. This may be demonstrated by immunofluorescence of hepatitis B antigen. Ig M and complements in the vessel wall would strongly suggest the role of the immunological phenomenon in the pathogenesis of this disease.

Hairy cell leukaemia can be indolent, and one quarter of patients present without significant symptoms or complications of the disease. These patients require no immediate therapy. Common infection includes legionella, toxoplasmosis, TB and atypical mycobacterial disease, nocardiasis and pyogenic infections. Since legionella is common in these patients, erythromycin should be administered to patients with pulmonary infiltrate. Therapy is directed with leukaemic patients with pancytopenia, recurrent infections and symptomatic splenomegaly, autoimmune complications or disease progressions. Splenectomy should not be performed except when life-threatening cytopenias must be corrected immediately.

The drugs which are highly active in inducing remission in hairy cell leukaemia are alpha interferon, deoxycoformycin (pentostatin) and 2-chlorodeoxyadenosine (2-CDA). Almost all patients respond to alpha interferon with 70% achieving major haematological benefits. Complete remission is rare, but treatment of recurrent disease is often successful. Short courses of glucocorticoids may be useful in controlling the vasculitis or the autoimmune manifestations that are often associated with hairy cell leukaemia, but not indicated as primary therapy. G-CSF may be used during neutropenic periods. The prognosis for hairy cell leukaemia is excellent.

Q 023

A young Eurasian couple returned from their honeymoon in Africa. They enjoyed an interesting safari, but had protracted diarrhoea. A fortnight after their return, their knees, ankles and fingers were extremely painful and swollen. They had pyrexia, myalgia and the wife developed bruises on her shins and face. The man has painful eyes.

A. What are the three possible diagnoses?
Ans: Post-infective reactive arthritis, Reiter's syndrome (post dysentery) and Dengue fever.

Tropical infections are common and patients leaving the UK should take advice from the London School of Tropical Medicine and Hygiene as different parts of the world expose them to exotic infections.

B. What three tests would you perform?
Ans: Joint aspiration, stool culture and blood culture.

C. How would you treat them?
Ans: I would initiate non-steroidal anti-inflammatory drugs, bed rest and medication for the husband as it may be anterior uveitis associated with Reiter's Syndrome.

Q 024

A 35-year-old widow had vaginal discharge, backache and pain on micturation. She was treated with a course of antibiotics, but did not comply with the therapy. Her symptoms improved, but she developed a rash 48 hours after taking the ampicillin. Ten days later she noticed pain and swelling in her left knee. She did not seek medical attention and she had an accident while cycling several days ago. The pain increased and she felt unwell. She attended her general practitioner who arranged an admission into the hospital.

On examination, she was febrile, temperature 103°F. Her left knee was hot, tender and swollen. She was admitted for investigation and treatment and discharged feeling well several weeks later. Several years later she complained of pain and stiffness of her hands, knee and feet. She was started on non-steroidal anti-inflammatory drugs and improved. She remained well for some years and was treated for depression as she became overly anxious about losing her job.

At the beginning of the year, she complained of dry cough which seemed to worsen in the evening and when she was climbing stairs. There was also breathlessness. The cough did not respond to antibiotics. Her condition deteriorated and she complained of unsteadiness and increasing weakness. She had difficulty in getting up from the chair without help and hence admitted to the hospital urgently.

On examination, she is pale and cyanosed. There is proximal myopathy and weakness. The joints of her hands are normal, but the skin is glossy and waxy in appearance. Her fingers are blue and tender. The pulse is regular at 70/min, blood pressure 150/130 mmHg, heart sounds are normal besides a pericardial friction rub is heard. In the lung, there are basal crackles.

Investigations:
- Hb – 10.7 g/dl
- WBC – 3 x 10^9/L
- ESR – 90 mm/hour
- Albumin – 24 g/L
- Globulin – 46 g/L
- Sodium – 135 mmol/L
- Potassium – 4.7 mmol/L
- Urea – 31 mmol/L
- LE test – negative
- ANF – positive

- Rheumatoid factor – positive
- Urine analysis showed albumin – +++
- WR – positive

A. What is the diagnosis of her initial illness?

Ans: Gonococcal arthritis and septicaemia.

Gonococcal rash often present with a few pustules. There is also a urinary infection with a septic rash. The rash with ampicillin suggests gonococcus.

B. Give three important investigations which should have been done on her initial admission?

Ans: Blood culture, endocervical swab, aspiration of knee joint for microscopy and culture.

The patient would have been treated with IV penicillin, spectinomycin or ciprofloxacin. Spectinomycin or ciprofloxacin should be considered if the rash is suspected to be an allergic reaction to penicillin.

C. What is the diagnosis of her present illness?

Ans: The different diagnoses are SLE, seleroderma (the skin and finger changes suggest the condition), mixed connective tissue disease, hypertension, arthritis, pericarditis and central nervous system involvement.

Q 025

A 31-year-old mother of three children is 38 weeks pregnant. Her 7-year-old child is recovering from a febrile illness. The mother is admitted with a vesicular rash and breathlessness.

A. What is the diagnosis?

Ans: Chicken pox (Varicella pneumonia)

B. The baby was delivered normally, but the mother was in great respiratory distress several days later. She was febrile and had malaise. There was an abnormal chest X-ray. What drug therapy should be started?

Ans: IV acyclovoir and the baby should be given zoster immunoglobulin plus IV acyclovir

C. How should the baby be managed in the first two weeks of life?
Ans: The baby is usually normal, but should be observed for the development of varicella. The mother's access to the child should be restricted until the lesions are crusted. The mother should be gowned, masked and gloved.

Q 026

A 9-year-old boy, a haemophiliac, gives a 3-day history of pain on the right side of his back. The pain is dull and keeps him awake at night, radiating to the right side of the abdomen and the groin, which persisted despite massive doses of analgesia. His mother treated him with cryoprecipitate (she works as a physician's assistant), but there was no obvious improvement. Three weeks ago he responded well to treatment for productive cough. He was diagnosed as having haemophilia when he was aged three, during a routine check-up. He suffers from frequent nose bleeds. There is no family history of a similar complaint. His father, who was studying for his USMLE gave factor VIII to the boy to which he temprorarily responded to.

On examination; he appears unwell and is in obvious pain. Pulse is 130/min; Blood pressure 110/70 mmHg; the heart sounds are normal and the lungs are clear. There is some tenderness in the right iliac fossa. His right hip is held in flexion and the extension of his right knee is painful and limited. There is reduced sensation over the anterior thigh of the right leg. The right knee jerk is absent.

Investigations:
- Hb – 9.3 g/dl
- MCV – 73 fl
- MCH – 22 picograms
- WBC – 11x 10^9/L
- Platelets – 210 x 10^9/L
- PIT – 70 sec

A. Give some cause for the failure to respond to treatment.
Ans:
i)   Insufficient quantity of factor VIII,
ii) Factor VIII given for insufficient time,

iii) Factor VIII inhibitors present in the patient's serum
iv) Poor quality factor VIII with low yield.

B. WHAT IS THE DIAGNOSIS?
ANS: A psoas haematoma which is compressing the femoral nerve, L3 and L4. He is anaemic because of the retroperitoneal bleed. The retroperitoneal haematoma may sometimes mimic malignant neoplasm - the pseudotumour syndrome.

Two of the most life-threatening sites of bleeding are in the oropharynx where the bleeding can compromise the airways and in the central nervous system. Intracerebral haemorrhage is one of the leading causes of death in patients with severe coagulation disorder.

Repeat joint bleeding may cause synovial thickening, chronic inflammation and fluid collection, and erode articular cartilage leading to joint deformities and limited mobility. Such deformities are particularly common in factor VIII and IX deficiency, the two sex-linked disorders referred to as haemophilia. For unclear reasons, haemarthrosis is much less common in other plasma coagulation disorders.

C. WHAT INVESTIGATIONS WOULD YOU PERFORM TO AID THE DIAGNOSIS?
ANS: An MRI or ultrasound to confirm the presence of a psoas haematoma. One could perform an assay for antibodies against factor VIII. The retroperitoneal haematoma caused femoral nerve compression.

Q 027

A 4-year-old is seen by her general practitioner because of vomiting, weight loss and constipation. She is the first born to a very successful period painter. Her birth weight was 3.6 kg. She has not been immunised and the mother is separated from the father. She is cared for by a nanny. The child and the father live in the studio flat. This is a decaying building in an ancient part of France. She has had upper respiratory tract infections frequently during the last six months, but has not been admitted to a hospital. She was prescribed some iron tablets by a local practitioner. On the evening of admission, she suddenly screamed and lost consciousness.

On examination, she is pale, undernourished and semiconscious. Temperature is 37°C. Head retraction and nucorigidity are present. The anterior frontanelle is closed. There is no cranial nerve or limb paralysis. The reflexes are all slowed and the plantar reflex is flexor. There is bilateral papilloedema observed and the pulse is 70/min, blood pressure 110/80 mmHg, no bruit is heard. The lungs and abdomen are normal.

Investigations:
- Hb – 7.5 g/dl
- WBC – 5.6 x 10⁹/L
- Blood sugar – 4 mmol/L
- Lumbar puncture (after a CT scan) showed 0.18×10^9 cells/L, 50% lymphocytes.
- Protein concentration – 1.56 g/L
- Glucose – 2.9 mmol/L
- Chloride – 91 mEq/L

A. What is the diagnosis?

Ans: The patient has lead encephalopathy as the reconstruction and the restoration of period painting may require lead. Diagnostic supporters are an increased delta amino levalunic acid, and an increased free erythrocyte protoporphyrin. The possibilities of TB meningitis should also be considered and the CFS should be stained with Ziehl Neelsen and cultured for tuberculosis.

In retrospect, a lumbar puncture should not have been performed. It is contraindicated if lead encephalopathy is present. A CT scan performed by an expert may demonstrate a lack of raised intracranial pressure by the size of the fourth ventricle.

In retrospect also, iron tablets should not have been given for anaemia as iron mobilises lead.

B. What investigations would you have performed to make a quick diagnosis?

Ans: An elevated serum lead level; the blood film may show basophilic stippling (punctate basophilia), microcytic hypochromic red blood cells, strongly positive quantitative urine corpoporphyrin.

The abdominal X-ray may demonstrate radiopaque signals that may represent recently ingested lead. The lead lines may be seen at the metaphysis of growing bone.

C. What are the principles of therapy for this patient?
Ans:
i)   To reduce cerebral oedema.
ii) The control and prevention of convulsions.
iii) The reduction of serum lead levels with BAL dimercaprol calcium edetate.

A 54-year-old engineer in London spent four months holidaying on the farm. He has been ill for the last three months, lost 8 kg in weight, and has a cough with white sputum. He has had night sweats, aching thigh muscles and a low backache. He is febrile, but has no lymphadenopathy. He is not jaundiced, the chest is clear and the liver is 4 cm below the right costal margin. The spleen is tender and 3 cm below the left costal margin.

- Hb – 13.6 g/L
- WBC – 3.6 x 10^9/L
- ESR – 70 mm/hour
- Chest X-ray is normal
- Blood culture x 6 – no growth

A. What is the most probable diagnosis?
Ans: Brucellosis.
    The other diagnoses to consider is lymphoma, but this is unlikely as the haemoglobin is normal and no lymph nodes are palpable. Tuberculosis is another possibility but the chest X-ray is normal.

B. How would you pursue the most likely diagnosis?
Ans: The definitive evidence of brucella infection consists of isolating the organism from the patient. Culturing brucella may be dangerous for laboratory personnel. Specimens should be labelled suspected brucellosis, and processed only in laboratories that have a biosafety level III facility. Up to 50% of untreated patients studied early in the course of infection will have brucella in the blood when a culture is grown in Tryticase soy broth for 1–3 nights in the presence of 10% carbon dioxide. Optimally Castemada medium (a biphasic trypticase soy broth) should be used

and incubated for four weeks.

Bone marrow cultures are often positive in acute brucellosis, whereas blood cultures are not. They are also more likely to remain positive later in the course of the disease in spite of the administration of antimicrobial agents. Only 20% of brucellosis cases are confirmed by a culture. In localised brucellosis, biopsy and isolation of brucella may be necessary for diagnosis. In a majority of cases of brucellosis, the diagnosis and isolation are made serologically. In brucellosis, most routine laboratory investigations are not helpful. The WBC is usually normal or low and the ESR may be normal.

There are four species of brucella that cause infection in humans. The most pathogenic is B. melitensis, followed by B. sius, B. abortus and B. canis. While each of these tend to produce infection in a specific animal host, B. melitensis in sheep and goats, B. sius in swine, B. abortus in cattle and B. canis in dogs, cross-species infection occurs eg. With B. abortus in sheep, and other animals can become infected too.

C. How would you treat if the diagnosis is confirmed?

Ans: The combination of doxycycline 100 mg every 12 hours or tetracycline 30 mg/kg/day in four equally divided doses orally for 3–6 weeks, plus streptomycin 50 mg/kg every 12 hours IM for the first four weeks is considered the treatment of choice.

Tetracycline should not be used in pregnant women and children because of the danger of staining developing teeth. Streptomycin may cause 8th nerve toxicity and the dose should be decreased in patients with renal insufficiency. An abscess should be drained when indicated.

Splenectomy has been performed in some patients with splenomegaly and multiple relapse and has apparently been successful in preventing a relapse. Splenectomy should not be performed until a high dose antimicrobial regimen has been attempted. Headache, backache and generalised aches and pains should be treated with analgesics.

Prognosis: Even before the advent of antimicrobial therapy, the mortality rate of brucellosis was less than 5% and only 15% had an illness exceeding three months in duration. With chemotherapy, the mortality rate is less than 2% and long illnesses and complications are rare. When the morbidity exceeds two months, other causes such as a previously unsuspected underlying disease or complications of brucellosis should be considered.

Q 029

A 17-year-old boy develops a sore throat and cough. He has been on phenytoin for epilepsy which started one month ago. On examination, he is febrile and there are white follicles on the tonsils and petechiae in the hard palate. Tender cervical occipital nodes are palpable in the neck. His GP treated him with penicillin, but this was stopped after 36 hours as he developed a generalised allergic rash. He made an uneventful recovery and was able to go hiking with his school mates. Two weeks after he returned from France, he felt unwell, began to lose weight and appetite. Apart from the nodes previously palpable, there were no abnormal clinical signs. He was treated with vitamin supplements, but did not improve. Six weeks later, he complained of night sweats, severe headache, productive cough with mucoid sputum and shortness of breath on exertion.

On examination, he is pale and looks ill. His gums are tender, swollen and bleed easily. Lymph nodes are palpable in the neck, axilla and groin. Both shins are tender with some raised purple zones. The heart, lungs and central nervous system are normal. The spleen is palpable in the abdomen.

Investigations:
- Hb – 10 g/dl
- WBC – 3 x 10^9/L
- Platelets – 110,000/mm^3
- CXR – bilateral hilar lymphadenopathy

A. WHAT IS THE LIKELIEST DIAGNOSIS AND WHAT ARE THE OTHER POSSIBLE DIAGNOSES?
ANS: The likeliest diagnosis for his condition is lymphoma. However, other diagnoses such as tuberculosis, aleukemic leukaemia, sarcoidosis and phenytoin induced pseudolymphoma need to be excluded.

B. WHAT IS THE POSSIBLE DIAGNOSIS FOR HIS INITIAL ILLNESS?
ANS: Infectious mononucleosis or streptococcal pharyngitis or penicillin allergy.

C. WHAT USEFUL INVESTIGATIONS WOULD YOU PERFORM?
ANS: A blood film, a lymph node biopsy and a bone marrow biopsy.

Q 030

A 6-year-old has growth retardation. He has a bloated abdomen and hepatomegaly.

Investigations revealed:
- Fasting glucose – 2.1 mmols/L
- Uric acid – 0.5 mmols/L
- Total Cholesterol – 12 mmols/L

A. WHAT IS THE DIAGNOSIS?

ANS: Von Gierke's disease. (Type I)

This is a glycogen-storage secondary to glucose 6 phosphatase deficiency. This is an autosomal recessive disorder. The patients are generally short and hyperglycaemia may produce convulsions in childhood. The kidneys are enlarged, a Fanconi like syndrome where phosphaturia is present. Renal insufficiency is associated with moderate proteinurua with focal and segmental glomerulosclerosis. Hyperurecaemia may cause gout. The kidneys and liver are uniformly enlarged.

B. WHAT INVESTIGATIONS WOULD YOU PERFORM TO CONFIRM THE DIAGNOSIS?

ANS: An infusion of glucagon would not increase the glucose. A liver biopsy would show deficiency of the enzyme glucose-6-phosphatase.

Q 031

A 40-year-old lady has lethargy, constipation, amenorrhoea, galactorrhoea and anaemia. She also complains of bumping into things and having difficulty with her sight. She was treated with thyroxine for two months, following which she became increasingly confused, suffered from abdominal pain, vomiting and collapsed one day.

Investigations:
- Thyroxine (T_4) – 35 nanomols/L
- TSH – 2 mU/L
- LH – 2 mU/L
- FSH – 2.1 mU/L
- Estradiol – 26 nanomols/L

A. What is the most likely diagnosis?
Ans: Hypopituitarism secondary to a pituitary tumour (is the commonest cause).

B. How would you confirm the diagnosis?
Ans: Combined triple pituitary stimulation test. MRI scan of the pituitary/ High resolution CT scan of the pituitary fossa.

C. What is the cause of her symptoms following thyroxine therapy?
Ans: Iatrogenic Addison's disease.
The thyroxine increases the basal metabolic rate and associated reduction of ACTH results in iatrogenic Addison's. In other words, increased metabolism of thyroxine has exarcebated the secondary hypoadrenalism, therefore corticotropin deficiency must be treated first.

Q 032

A 43-year-old man is admitted with acute left hemiplegia. He is noted to be passing dark red urine and has been treated for two episodes of deep vein thrombosis in the past, but is not on any medication currently.

Investigations:
- Hb – 8 g/dl
- WBC – 3.6 x 10^9/L
- Platelets – 60 x 10^9/L
- Reticulocyte count – 1%
- Blood film – Normal (some hypersegmentation is seen)
- Coomb's test – negative

A. What is the diagnosis?
Ans: Aplastic anaemia as a complication of paroxysmal nocturnal haemoglobunuria. This is not an autoimmune form of pancytopenia. A different diagnosis is paroxysmal cold haemoglobinaemia.

Q 033

A 6-year-old Gypsy boy was brought in by his father because he thought the son was not growing and his leg appeared odd. He said both he and the mother were short. His other son, age eight, was 128 cm tall.

On examination he looked well, height 90 cm, weight 18 kg. There was bowing of his legs, but there were no other abnormalities.

Investigations:
- Full blood count, ESR, urea, electrolytes and blood sugar were all normal.
- Calcium – 2.12 mmol/L
- Phosphates – 0.21 mmol/L
- Alkaline phosphatase – 160 IU/L (Normal range between 25–28 IU/L)
- X-ray Wrist – metaphysis split and cut. The epiphyses were widened. The growth plates were widened. He was referred to the hospital for further management and was treated with vitamin D. One year later his height was 91 cm.

Investigations:
- Serum calcium – 2.2 mmol/L
- Phosphate – 0.32 mmol/L
- Alkaline phosphatase – 135 IU/L
- X-ray wrist – Previous changes have almost resolved.

A. WHAT IS THE UNDERLYING DIAGNOSIS?
ANS: This child has familial hypophosphataemic rickets and should be treated with oral phosphates.

X-linked hypophosphataemia, also called vitamin D resistance rickets, is an X-linked dominant disorder. The rate of linear growth is at first normal and then slowed. In some patients, spontaneous remission may be followed by recurrence in adult life, eg. during pregnancy and lactation.

An autosomal recessive disease, the adult Fanconi syndrome occurs in the absence of any systemic disorder. The term 'adult' is misleading because the cases are recognised in childhood, but no apparent abnormalities are present at birth. Dwarfism and hypophophataemic rickets occur with the laboratory anomalies of Fanconi syndrome. Renal failure is rare and the prognosis is good when the systemic manifestations are treated.

B. WHAT CONDITIONS APPEAR TO BE TRANSMITTED BY THIS MODE OF INHERITANCE?

ANS: X-linked dominant traits include the Xg (a+) blood group. Some rare conditions may be inherited in X-linked dominant traits in which there is manifestation of the condition in the hemizygous male. The characteristics of this form of inheritance are demonstrated by predigree charts.

The disorder occurs only in females who are heterozygous for the mutant gene and the affected mothers transmit to half their daughters and an increased frequency of abortion occurs in the affected women. The abortions occurs in affected male foetuses.

Conditions that appear to be transmitted by this mode of transmission include *incontinentia pigmenti*, local dermal hypoplasia, oral–fascial-digital syndrome and hyperammonemia due to ornithine transcarbamylase deficiency.

Q 034

A 14-year-old boy has a history of recurrent nose-bleed since he was 6 years old.

Investigation:
- Bleeding time – 16 min
- Prothrombin time – 13.5 sec (control – 13.4 sec)
- Partial thromboplastin time – 55 sec (control – 34 sec)
- HESS test – positive
- Hb – 8 g/dl
- WBC – 7.7 x 10^9/L
- Platelets – 210 x 10^9/L

A. WHAT IS THE LIKELY DIAGNOSIS?
ANS: Von Willebrand's disease.

B. WHAT INVESTIGATIONS WOULD HELP TO CONFIRM THE DIAGNOSIS?
ANS: Factor VIII levels and related antigens. Both would be depressed.

C. IS GENETIC COUNSELLING AND CARRIER DETECTION FEASIBLE IN THIS CONDITION?
ANS: Carrier detection requires a biologic and immunological assay

which compares the ratio of factor VIII to the von Willebrand's factor protein and is predictive only up to 80% of cases. It is now possible to trace the defective allele by examining the inheritance of restriction fragment-length polymorphism (RFLPs) linked to the factor VIII genes. Factors with specific mutation have been defined in the factor VIII gene. This can be readily detected by gene amplification and allele-specific oligonuclotide hybridisation.

Previous prenatal diagnostic techniques required foetal blood for coagulant activity. Now, in families with identifiable RFLP linked to the gene or known mutation, precise diagnosis is possible in early pregnancy for either chorionic villus biopsy or amniocentesis. The amount of sample required has decreased and the speed of the diagnosis has increased with the introduction of the PCR technique (polymerase chain reaction) to amplify the desired segment of the genomic DNA.

Female carriers of haemophilia, who are heterozygous, usually produce sufficient factor VIII from the factor VIII allele on their normal X chromosomes for normal haemostasis. However, occasionally haemophilia carriers have factor VIII levels far below 50% due to random inactivation of affected IX chromosomes in tissue-producing factor VIII. These symptomatic carriers may bleed with major surgery or bleed occasionally with menses. Rarely, true female haemophiliacs arise from consanguinity within families with haemophilia or from concomitant Turner's syndrome or XO mosaicism in a female carrier.

Q 035

A 26-year-old bus conductor is investigated for impotence. His friends have commented that his skin has become more tanned over the last eight months.

Investigations:
- Testosterone – 5 mmol/L (normal 14 – 42 mmol/L)
- Prolactin – 355 IU/L (normal less than 450 IU/L)
- Thyroxine – 67 mmol/L
- FSH – 2.1 units/L (normal 3–8 units/L)
- LH – 3.4 units/L (normal 3–8 units/L)
- Insulin tolerance test (0.15 units of insulin/Kg after 30 min – 0)
  - Glucose 5 mmol/L at 2 min

- Glucose hormone test MU/L 4 at 20 min
- Cortisol mmol/L – 600 at 120 min

A. WHAT IS THE DIAGNOSIS?

ANS: This patient has hypogonadotropic hypogonadism.

This condition occurs both in men and women due to iron deposition in the pituitary. Tissue injury may result from destruction of iron laden lysosomes, from lipid peroxidation of subcellular organelles by excess iron or stimulation of collagen synthesis by the excess iron. The etiology of the condition in this case is haemochromatosis.

In 1989, Von Recklinghausen named the disease 'haemochromatosis' and the iron storage pigment 'haemosiderin' because he believed the pigment was derived from the blood. Haemochromatosis implies the presence of potential severe progressive iron overload leading to fibrosis and organ failure.

Cirrhosis, diabetes mellitus, arthritis, cardiomyopathy and hypogonadotropic hypogonadism are the usual manifestations. The disease is due to the inheritance of a mutant gene that is tightly linked to HLA-6 locus on the short arm of chromosome 6. Acquired haemochromatosis may also occur, secondary to an iron overloading state such as thalassaemia or sideroblastic anaemia. Porphyria cutanea tarda (PCT), a disorder characterised by a defect in prophyrin biosynthesis, is also sometimes associated with excessive parenchymal iron deposition. However, the magnitude of iron load is usually inadequate to produce tissue damage. The exact relationship between these two diseases is unclear, although iron may accentuate the inherited enzyme deficiency in PCT. Haemochromatosis in heavy drinkers may be distinguished from alcoholic liver disease by two means:

i) Measurement of hepatic iron concentration.
ii) Studying relatives for evidence of the disease, including HLA typing.

Excessive iron ingestion over many years, if ever, results in clinical, as well as pathological, haemochromatosis. One important exception are South African Blacks (Bantu) - their intake of excessive iron in an alcoholic beverage is due to the practice of brewing fermented beverages in vessels made out of iron.

B. Is there any advantage in the diet of the South African Bantu tribe?

Ans: The ingestion of high iron predisposes to haemochromatosis, but their diet rich in roughage produces bulky stools. Therefore, they have a lower incidence of large bowel cancers compared to their American and Europeans counterparts. Dietary fibres accelerate intestinal transmission time, reducing the exposure time of the colonic mucosa to potential carcinogens, and diluting these carcinogens because of increasing fecal bulk.

There has been a similar observation in Seventh-day Adventists who are vegetarians. A diet low in fibres leads to constipation and diverticulosis. There is a problem in this hypothesis. If a low fibre diet alone is a significant factor in colorectal cancers, individuals having diverticulosis should be at a higher risk for developing large bowel tumours. This does not appear to be the case.

Q 036

A 45-year-old farmer has a cough of 8-days duration. He is treated with amoxycillin. He develops nausea, vomiting, anorexia, and the antibiotic is stopped. He is admitted to the hospital and is found to be jaundiced. His stool is pale, but the urine is dark. His liver is palpable, smooth and slightly tender, 4 cm below the costal margin. Five years ago he received a right hemicolectomy for carcinoma of the colon. He does not smoke and drinks alcohol socially.

Investigations:
- Hb – 15 g/dl
- WBC – 9 x 10^9 /L
- Platelets – 140 x 10^9/L
- ESR – 5
- Bilirubin – 60 micromol/L
- Alkaline phophatase – 145 IU/L
- AST – 66 IU/L (normally less than 30 IU/L)
- ALT – 96 IU/L (normally less than 35 IU/L)
- Hepatitis B surface antigen screen – negative

Five days later, he feels better and returns home, but is readmitted after a

week as he felt tired and nauseated. The investigations reveal:
- Hb – 15 g/dl
- ESR – 2
- Bilirubin – 29 minicromol/L
- Alkaline phosphatase – 130 IU/L
- AST – 62 IU/L
- ALT – 118 IU/L
- Sodium – 140 mmol/L
- Potassium – 4 mmol/L
- Urea – 5 mmol/L

A. WHAT ARE THE MOST LIKELY DIAGNOSIS?
ANS: Hepatitis A, Q fever, alcoholic hepatitis and mycoplasma pneumonia.

The obvious diagnosis is hepatitis A. Alcoholic hepatitis is a possibility as the condition improves in the hospital, recurring on discharge. The whole episode is too short for chronic hepatitis and one must evoke another cause for infective hepatitis. Infectious mononucleosis is a possibility and should be considered.

Leptospirosis is also a possibility although the patient would be more seriously ill and there would be other signs (and this can easily be excluded by a leptospirosis IgM test). Q fever often starts with a respiratory infection and one-third of patients develops acute or chronic hepatitis, although only 10% are jaundiced. Mycoplasma occasionally gives rise to hepatitis.

B. APART FROM A LIVER BIOPSY, NAME A TEST WHICH WILL HELP DISTINGUISH BETWEEN THE DIFFERENT DIAGNOSES.
ANS: Cold agglutinin. Serology would not be the correct answer.

Cold agglutinin would be compatible for mycoplasma, and a raised gamma glutamyl transferase would support the diagnosis of alcoholism. Acute hepatitis A may be supported by the the presence of IgM to anti HAV. Q fever may be supported by antibodies to *coxiella burnetii*.

Q 037

A 36-year-old woman is admitted for investigation and treatment of hypertension. She is found to be hypertensive and is started on thiazide diuretics and methyldopa 250 mg BD, but this did not bring down hypertension towards the end of her first pregnancy 12 years ago. There is no history of hypertension and she does not smoke or drink alcohol. Her husband is an engineer and spends a great deal of time away from home. He has been under considerable financial strain and drinks heavily.

On examination, the blood pressure is 230/ 130 mmHg, the fundi demonstrates mild hypertensive changes with arterio-venous nipping. The cardiovascular and respiratory system is normal. Urine analysis reveal trace proteins, but no blood. Microscopy is normal. She is started on a small dose of bendrofluazide and ACE inhibitor. Three weeks later, she complains of lethargy, that she is unable to stand from a kneeling position while praying in the Buddhist temple. While her blood pressure was being recorded, she develops tetanic spasms which appear to be acute abnormal writhing movements to the layman and they are worried that she may be possessed.

A. What is the cause of her tetany?
Ans: Low ionized calcium with hypokalaemia as she was hyperventilating.

B. What is the cause of her inability to get to her feet while she was in the Buddist temple?
Ans: Hypokalaemia.

C. What is the diagnosis?
Ans: Conn's syndrome and spironolactone will control her symptoms while waiting for lab results.

Q 038

A 43-year-old chemistry teacher had a routine chest X-ray which revealed bilateral hilar lymphadenopathy. He is asymptomatic except for a violaceous rash on his chest. He has a medical history of hepatitis A which was resolved, and there are no findings on examination.

A. What are the possible diagnoses?
Ans: Sarcoidosis, lymphoma, leukaemia and tuberculosis. The cutaneous

changes may be the manifestation of sarcoidosis on the skin, also called lupus pernio.

Q 039

A 43-year-old hair designer has had a gradual increase in breathlessness and a dry cough, which he explains away as smoker's cough, for the last six weeks. He has had pain in his left elbow and ankles, and feels generally unwell. He had no significant history except sniffing cocaine occasionally which he has not done for the last eight months.

The ECG and chest X-ray are normal and echocardiography did not reveal any abnormalities. He is well physically, but blood gases reveal a PO_2 8.1 and PCO_2 of 5 KPa.

A. WHAT IS THE DIAGNOSIS?
ANS: Pneumocystis carini pneumonia secondary to immunosuppression.

This is suggested by his dry cough, dyspnoea and hypoxia. In such cases the chest X-ray is usually normal, but at times one may find a perihilar flare.

B. WHAT INVESTIGATIONS SHOULD BE PERFORMED?
ANS: The patient should have a CD4 count. A bronchioalveolar lavage should be performed and stained with Grocot's stain (silver stain) to search for pneumocystis carinii.

The patient should undergo HIV test after counselling. If the test is positive, the patient should be treated with a protease inhibitor and AZT. The pneumocystis carinii pneumonia should be treated with cotrimoxazole. Nebulised pentamidine may be used and one may also consider the combination of dapsone and trimethoprim.

The application of high dose steroids has been suggested as this may reduce interstitial fibrotic changes. It is now considered medical malpractice if one does not include HAART (Highly Active Antiretroviral Therapy). This has been shown to increase the longevity of the patient.

Q 040

A 45-year-old prostitute develops severe pain behind her ear while walking the streets. Fifteen minutes later she vomits and the pain lessens to some extent, but she has to stay in bed in a flat which she shares with two women. She registers double vision with horizontal separation of images when she looks to the left, shortly after the incident in the street. Her pimp comments that her right eyelid is drooping and tells her she should cut down on the codeine that she is drinking.

On examination there is slight ptosis on the right side with limitation of adduction, elevation and depression of the right eye. The pupil is dilated and unresponsive to light when light is shone into both eyes. The 5th nerve is intact and there are no significant signs except a raised BP of 180/90 mmHg. Her symptoms improved for 2–3 days, but she is then admitted as an emergency case when she is found unconscious on the curb.

A. What is the diagnosis?

Ans: This patient has a posterior communicating artery aneurysm which had caused a 3rd nerve palsy and a sub-arachnoid haemorrhage.

Pain in and behind the eye in the lower temple can occur with an expanding middle cerebral artery aneurysm. A sudden and unexplainable headache at any location should raise suspicion of a subarachnoid bleed and should be investigated by CT scan to look for blood in the basal system. Often a small subarachnoid haemorrhage will not be seen by a CT scan and a lumbar puncture should be performed to detect the presence of blood.

Third nerve palsy, when associated with pupillary dilation, loss of light reflex and focal pain in and behind the eye, indicates an expanding aneurysm at the junction of the posterior communicating artery and the internal carotid artery. Early surgery is indicated.

B. Where would you consider the lesion to be if the 6th nerve is involved?

Ans: I would consider a lesion in the cavernous sinus.

Visual field defects can occur with an expanding supraclinoid aneurysm. Occipital and posterior cervical pain may signal a posteroinferior cerebellar artery (PICA) or an anteroinferior cerebellar artery (AICA) aneurysm.

C. WHAT WOULD YOU CONSIDER IF THE PATIENT HAD 3RD NERVE PALSY WITH PUPILLARY SPARING? (PUPILLARY SPARING MEANS NORMAL SIZE AND NORMAL REFLEX RESPONSE)

ANS: This suggests an isolated, painful 3rd nerve palsy, due to a microinfarct caused by diabetes mellitus, hypertension or collagen vascular disease.

Patients over age 50 with an isolated 3rd nerve palsy and pupil sparing without signs of subarachnoid haemorrhage have a better prognosis. Recovery following microinfarction of the nerve is usually complete within 3 months. In the absence of recovery, the patient should be investigated.

Q 041

A 25-year-old sailor from Port au Spain was ill at sea with fever and headache. He was well in the past, but has had periods of an unexplained cough for two years, not severe and resolved spontaneously. Four members of his immediate family have had tuberculosis.

On examination, he has a temperature of 38.4°C and a stiff neck. The left optic disc is normal, but the left is not adequately visualised as there is some cloudiness in the anterior chamber. There is bilateral parotid enlargement and the liver and spleen are palpably enlarged. He has no focal neurology apart from facial weakness which affects the lower and upper face.

A. WHAT ARE THE POSSIBILITIES?

ANS: One should consider the possibility of sarcoidosis, a systemic disease which almost always affects the lungs.

The combination of bilateral parotid enlargement and 7th nerve palsy is a variety of sarcoidosis known as the uveoparotid syndrome. The Melkerson-Rosenthal syndrome comprises a rare triad of recurrent and eventually permanent facial paralysis, recurrent and eventually permanent facial (labial) oedema and less constantly plication of the tongue.

Tuberculosis must be considered as he has had contact with close family members. Lymphoma may present itself in the manner described above.

B. HOW ELSE WOULD YOU INVESTIGATE THIS PATIENT?
ANS: I would perform a lumbar puncture after an MRI or a CT scan. A tissue biopsy may be obtained from the liver and spleen after the bleeding time and the platelet count have been measured.

C. HOW WOULD YOU EXPLAIN THE OCULAR INVOLVEMENT?
ANS: The eye is involved in one quarter of patients with sarcoidosis and this may lead to blindness. The usual lesion involves the uveal tract, iris, ciliary body and the choroid. Seventy-five percent have anterior uveitis and up to 35% have posterior uveitis. There is blurred vision, tearing and photophobia. The uveitis may develop rapidly and clear spontaneously over 6–12 months. It may also develop insidiously and become chronic. Conjunctival involvement is also common, usually with small, yellow nodules. When the lacrimal gland is involved, a keratoconjunctiva sicca syndrome with dry sore eyes may result.

Most cases of uveitis are idiopathic. Systemic diseases causing uveitis, apart from sarcoidosis, include psoriatic arthropathy, juvenile rheumatoid arthritis (rheumatoid factor negative), juvenile nevoxanthogranuloma, rheumatoid arthritis, Lyme's disease and relapsing polychondritis.

Treatment of uveitis include cycloplegics, glucocorticoids and immunosuppressive drugs such as chorambucil, azothioprine, cyclophosphamide and cyclosporin A.

Q 042

A 46-year-old football player has fatigue, back pain and, occasionally, shooting pain in the buttocks and the back of his legs. He smokes heavily and has minor attacks of bronchitis. There are no definite physical signs at that stage. Three days later, he notices tingling in both feet and weakness of the legs, a condition that becomes progressively worse over the next few days. He also notices weakness and clumsiness of his hands, and begins to have difficulty in passing urine.

On examination, the cranial nerves are normal. There are proximal and distal weaknesses in all four limbs and all the tendon reflexes are unobtainable. Both plantar reflexes are difficult to assess, but are thought to be extensors. Sensory examination is normal apart from the impairment of vibration appreciation in both feet.

A. WHAT IS THE MOST LIKELY DIAGNOSIS?
Ans: The Gullian-Barré syndrome.

B. WHAT OTHER POSSIBILITIES SHOULD BE CONSIDERED?
Ans: A compressive cord lesion because of the involvement of the bladder.

C. HOW SHOULD HE BE INVESTIGATED?
Ans: A CT scan, MRI or a myelogram.

Q 043

A 36-year-old alcoholic is admitted to the hospital in a confused and anxious state. He smells strongly of alcohol and has a cut over his right jaw. He has mild unsteadiness of gait and nystagmus in all directions of gaze. He is unable to stand and the ankle jerk cannot be elicited. The tone of the lower limbs is reduced. He has a *grand mal* epileptic seizure the next day, after which he is drowsy. Later in the day he is found in another ward in a restless and agitated state. He becomes increasingly difficult to communicate with, ranging from an agitated and confused state to one of drowsiness and immobility.

Formal examination is extremely difficult, but he appears to have some limitation of eye-movement and persistent nystagmus, as well as variable weakness in all four limbs.

A. WHAT IS THE MOST LIKELY DIAGNOSIS?
Ans: This patient has Wernicke - Korsakoff syndrome.

This is a medical emergency and requires immediate administration of thiamine. A delay of a few hours may be crucial in determining whether the patient with ocular and ataxic signs can be prevented from developing an amnestic state, and whether the patient with early Korsakoff changes will be restored to a state of mental competency. Three mg of thiamine may modify the ocular signs, and much larger doses are needed to replenish the thiamine stores. High dose IM or IV thiamine should be given every day until the patient resumes a normal diet. If the patient cannot or will not eat, parenteral feeding of Vitamin B is necessary.

Treating a patient with IV glucose infusion may deplete the patient's reserve of Vitamin B and can either cause Wernicke's encephalopathy or a rapid worsening form of the disease. Due to this, Vitamin B must be administered to alcoholics and patients requiring parenteral glucose.

The topography of the lesions produced by thiamine deficiency has been studied in rhesus monkeys. Witt and Goldman-Rakic found that the severity and the number of brain nuclei affected are related to the duration and number of bouts of thiamine deficiency.

Wernicke's encephalopathy normally develops in an orderly sequence, comprising vomiting, nystagmus, palsy of the recti muscles leading to uninateral or bilateral ophthalmoplegia, fever, ataxia and progressive mental deterioration that eventually results in global confusional states and coma. Improvement occurs after the administration of thiamine although Korsakoff s psychosis may intervene. Korsakoff's syndrome is characterised by retrograde amnesia, impaired ability to learn and confabulation.

In summary Wernicke's encephalopathy and the amnestic psychosis of the Korsakoff's syndrome are not separate clinical events. Instead they are difficult to differentiate as both develope ocular and ataxic signs, the transformation of the global confusion into amnesic confabulatory syndrome and the development of a non-confabulatory amnesic state are successive stages in the recovery from a single pathological process.

Diagnostic confirmation may be the clinical response after the administration of thiamine. In 1977 when Sudden Asian Cardiac death occurred frequently in Hmong refugees in America, Thai and Filipino workers in Singapore and Malaysia, thiamine deficiency and beri-beri were considered, but the culprit truned out to be the Brugada Syndrome. This is diagnosed easily on ECG.

Beri-beri is associated with an increase in blood pressure and a decrease in heart rate within 12 hours after commencing therapy, followed by diuresis and a reduction in heart size within 1–2 days. In untreated cases of Wernicke's disease, there is invariably an elevation of blood pyruvate and a reduction in the blood transketolase (thiamine dependant enzyme of the Hexose Monophosphate shunt). A diffuse slowing of the EEG, mild to moderate, occurs in 50% of patients.

Q 044

A 55-year-old lady, a pig farmer, is afflicted with malaise, weight loss, and weakness in all four limbs. The pain mainly affects her shoulders.

Investigations:
- Sodium – 142 mmols/L
- Potassium – 3.4 mmols/L
- Calcium – 2.35 mmols/L
- AST – 114 IU/L
- CPK – 180 U/L
- Hb – 9.7 g/dl
- ESR – 70 mm/h

A. WHAT IS THE MOST LIKELY DIAGNOSIS AND WHAT DIFFERENTIAL DIAGNOSIS WOULD YOU CONSIDER?
ANS: The most likely diagnosis is polymyositis, but the possibility of trichinella infection and muscular dystrophy must also be considered. As this patient is above 50, the possibility of an occult neoplasm must be considered. If the polymyositis is the result of an occult neoplasm, the polymyositis is a paraneoplastic manifestation.

The diagnosis of polymyositis may be clinched by EMG and muscle biopsy. One must be careful not to take the diagnosis from sites which have undergone recent venepuncture as this may simulate the histopathological picture. The presence of a rash with polymyositis is called dermatomyositis.

Q 045

A 28-year-old Indian swimming instructor is admitted with headache, neck stiffness and intermittent diplopia.

The CSF findings:
- Pressure – 22 cm of water
- RBC – 9/cubic mm
- WBC – 364/cubic mm (lymphocytes 70%, neutrophils 20%, monocytes 10%)
- Proteins – 80 mg/ 100 m1
- Glucose – 1.4 mmol/L

A. WHAT IS THE MOST LIKELY DIAGNOSIS?
ANS: The most likely diagnosis is TB meningitis. One should also consider syphilis, leukaemia and lymphoma.

Q 046

A 63-year-old washer woman presents with proximal muscle weakness and tingling in her left hand. The patient's friend noticed that she was jaundiced.

- Hb – 10 g/dl
- MCV – 100 fl
- Sodium – 125 mmol/L
- Potassium – 4.2 mmol/L
- Cholesterol – 8.6 mmol/L

A. WHAT IS THE DIAGNOSIS?
ANS: Hypothyroidism with carotenaemia.

B. WHAT OTHER THREE INVESTIGATIONS WILL CONFIRM THE DIAGNOSIS?
ANS: TSH, T_4 and EMG.

Q 047

A 3-year-old baby has convulsions.

- Blood glucose – 5.7 mmol/L
- Calcium – 1.2 mmo1/L
- Phosphate – 3.7 mmol/L
- Alkaline phosphatase – 130 IU/L
- Urea – 6.3 mmol/L

A. What is the most likely diagnosis?
Ans: Feed with cow's milk which contains a high level of phosphate.

Q 048

A 21-year-old medical student is afflicted with apathy, muscle stiffness and tremors of the hands. He has slurred speech and his writing has deteriorated. The urine test shows glycosuria.

- Sodium – 143 mmol/L
- Potassium – 2.6 mmol/L
- Bicarbonate – 12 mmol/L
- AST – 48 IU/L
- Bilirubin – 30 µmols/L
- Urea – 5.6 mmol/L
- Glucose – 5.1 mmol/L

A. WHAT OTHER PHYSICAL SIGNS WOULD YOU LOOK FOR?
ANS: The Kayser-Fleischer ring.

B. WHAT IS THE DIAGNOSIS?
ANS: This patient has Wilson's disease with proximal tubular acidosis.

Q 049

A 56-year-old man presented with a recent cough and is suffering from a progressive inability to stand, beginning with right leg weakness and now the left.

The CSF:
- Pressure – 130 mm of water
- RBC – 3/cubic mm
- WBC – 3 mononuclear cells
- Protein – 264 mg/ 100 ml
- Glucose – 4 mmol/L (blood – 5.3 mmol/L)

A. WHAT ARE THE POSSIBLE EXPLANATIONS OF THESE FINDINGS?
ANS: Guillian-Barré syndrome, Legionaire's disease, lymphoma and the paraneoplastic syndrome.

Q 050

A 43-year-old Jamaican singer has headache and progressive visual failure. His blood pressure on admission is 220/140 mmHg.

A. What is the most likely diagnosis?
Ans: Malignant hypertension.

B. Why does he have hypokalaemia?
Ans: Secondary hyperaldosteronism due to diuretics.

C. What other possible diagnoses would you consider?
Ans: A pituitary tumour, cranial meningioma, Paget's disease and temporal arteritis.

Q 051

A 23-year-old trainee pilot with Crohn's disease has tingling in his hands and tetany. He does not appear to be over-breathing.

Investigation:
- Sodium – 141 mmol/L
- Potassium – 3.1 mmol/L
- Bicarbonate – 26 mmol/L
- Calcium – 2.1 mmol/L
- Phosphate – 0.85 mmol/L
- Albumin – 27 g/L

A. What is the explanation?
Ans: This patient has hypomagnesemia. Hypomagnesemia may also be a consequence of therapy with aminoglycosides, cisplatinum and diuretics.

Q 052

A 26-year-old architect has arthralgia, a facial rash, headache and disturbance of mood. She has been behaving abnormally and appears to have paranoid delusions. She lost her temper this morning and had to be restrained when she struck a co-worker with a shovel. Shortly after admission, she had a generalised seizure.

The blood results:
- Hb – 9.8 g/dl

- WBC – 3.8 x 10^9/L
- Platelet – 85 x 10^9/L
- Urea – 14.5 mmol/L

A. WHAT IS THE MOST LIKELY DIAGNOSIS?
ANS: SLE

B. WHAT OTHER NEUROLOGICAL COMPLICATIONS COULD ARISE?
ANS: Mononeuritis multiplex, cerebrovascular accident and chorea. Studies from Hong Kong have suggested that many cases of SLE in Asia are complicated by cerebral TB.

Q 053

A baby has a history of fits, all of which occurred in the early morning, waking both the parents. He is found to have a large liver.

- Fasting glucose – 2.1 mmol/L
- AST – 18 IU/L
- Alkaline phosphatase – 170 IU/L
- Bilirubin – 13 micromol/L
- Urea – 0.78 mmol/L

A. WHAT IS THE CAUSE OF THE FITS AND WHAT IS THE EXPLANATION FOR THE ALKALINE PHOSPHATASE?
ANS: This patient has Von Gierke's disease.

The alkaline phophatase is raised as the child is growing. This patient should undergo a liver biopsy and have an enzyme assay performed.

Q 054

A 65-year-old man is admitted for investigation of back pain, malaise and weight loss. He has signs of peripheral neuropathy suggested by glove and stocking anaesthesia.

- Hb – 11 g/d1
- ESR – 80 mm/h
- Calcium – 2.7 mmol/L

- Albumin – 30 g/L
- The nerve conduction studies show motor and sensory neuropathy with a slight slowing in the conduction velocity.

A. What are the possible diagnoses?
Ans: One should consider myeloma, carcinoma and sarcoidosis.

Q 055

A 63-year-old man develops difficulties in his work as a medical superintendent. His speech tends to falter and he has a problem searching for the right words, a failure of memory with things he would normally remember and a great difficulty with any work involving simple arithmetic. These symptoms had come on insidiously and he has deteriorated gradually over the last four months. He is right handed.

On examination, he is alert and intelligent, but his speech is hesitant and he has difficulty in naming common objects. Mental arithmetic is poorly performed and he is unable to remember a name and address after five minutes. Fundoscopy reveals the optic disc is normal, but there is no visible venous pulsation. He has an upper quadrant field defect on the right side, which is homonymous and confluent. There is lower facial weakness on the right side. The left ear is deaf and there is weakness and sensory impairment in the limbs, but the tendon reflexes are slightly brisker on the right, with an extensor plantar respond on the same side.

A. Where is the lesion?
Ans: The left temporal lobe.

B. What are the possible pathological diagnoses?
Ans: Abcesses, tumour (such as glioma, meningioma or metastasis), bronchogenic carcinoma with secondaries in the brain.

C. How should this patient be investigated and treated?
Ans: A CT scan or an MRI of the brain.

Q 056

A 25-year-old musician has pins and needles in both feet. He complains of a tight feeling around his left leg like a bandage. His left leg feels faintly weak and drags when he is tired. He noticed an urgency of micturation and deterioration of potency for six weeks. He has to bend his head fully forward or backwards at work. He had noticed when he bends his head forward or backward, he has tingling sensations in his back and legs. He has been well, apart from an episode of vertigo three years ago, diagnosed to be viral labarynthitis.

On examination, there is no abnormal finding in the cranial nerves and the upper limbs. The tone is increased in both legs and there is mild weakness in the left leg. Both the knee and ankle jerks are brisk and the plantar responses were ellicted in the right leg. Position sensation was abnormal in both feet, more so in the left. There is a positive Lhermitte sign.

A. What is the diagnosis?
Ans: Multiple sclerosis with a plaque involving the left side of the spinal cord. One must also consider an acute disc prolapse and a neurofibroma.

B. What investigation should be performed?
Ans: An MRI, visual evoked response. EP studies may detect and localise lesions in afferent pathways in the central nervous system. They have been used to investigate patients with suspected multiple sclerosis, the diagnosis of which requires the recognition of lesions involving several regions of the central white matter. In patients with suspected multiple sclerosis (or other neurological disorders) and with vague and ill-defined complaints, the organic basis of symptoms may be supported by the presence of EP abnormalities in the appropriate afferent pathway. MRI is helpful in detecting lesions in patients with multiple sclerosis, but electrophysiology studies are cheaper and monitor the functional rather than the anatomical status of the afferent pathway under study.

One should perform an MRI of the spinal cord to screen for a prolapse and neurofibroma. Visual and auditory acuity can be determined by an ophthalmologist and an audiologist using EP technique if a patient's age or mental state precludes his/her co-operation for behavioural testing.

Q 057

A 55-year-old butcher develops a transient numbness and clumsiness of the right hand while at work, with a tingling sensation on the right side of the face. The symptoms resolved completely within 10 minutes, but he had a second, more prolonged episode over the next three days. On that occasion, the symptoms lasted 20 minutes and he was aware of difficulty in his speech during the attack. He has a history of myocardial infarction two years ago and still smokes 30 cigarettes a day. He recalls two episodes when he suddenly lost vision in his left eye, lasting less than 30 seconds on each occasion.

On examination, there are no abnormal neurological signs. He is in sinus rhythm with a heart rate of 100/min and his blood pressure is 160/100 mmHg. The heart sounds are normal. There is short systolic bruit on both sides of the neck. The superficial temporal pulse is difficult to feel on the right side.

A. WHAT IS THE DIAGNOSIS?

ANS: Transient ischaemic attack involving the middle cerebral artery.

He should be investigated with a carotid Doppler. With a competent circle of Willis, the occlusion can be entirely asymptomatic. Arteriosclerosis in the proximal internal carotid artery is usually more severe in the Iˢᵗ 2cm and they arise from the posterior wall, often extending downward to the common carotid artery.

This patient complains of mono-ocular blindness (*amaurosis fugax*). Non-stenotic or slightly stenotic lesions in conjunction with a stroke or a single prolonged TIA suggest the heart is the source of the embolus.

Atheromatous lesions at the origin of the great vessels in the aortic arch also produce cerebral emboli that can cause transient ischaemia or infarction, but the incidence of this mechanism is low. When a major carotid territory stroke is suspected, the middle cerebral artery stem (*Lenticulostriae*) and peripheral (cortical surface) territory may both be infarcted. In this setting, acute anticoagulation is avoided because preventing further stroke is not an issue and haemorrhage into the lenticulostriae territory is a possible complication.

Heparin prevents clot propagation and formation by potentiating anti-thrombin III activity. Heparin therapy is sometimes advocated when a tightly stenotic internal carotid artery or an impending or complete carotid or middle cerebral artery occlusion is suspected.

Carotid endarterectomy should only be considered if the stenosis is more than 70% and after the patient is stabilised.

B. How should this patient be treated if he has critical involvement of the carotid artery and critical coronary artery disease requiring coronary artery bypass grafting?

Ans: Both surgical procedures should be performed at the same time. This has been demonstrated to reduce mortality and morbidity.

Q 058

A 53-year-old parachute instructor has muscle weakness and fatigue. His symptoms are rather vague, but he describes difficulty walking. He feels giddy as he jumps from the plane, his shoulder muscle feels weak and he has a problems getting up from the ground. He has lost weight and has headaches, aches in the lower back and a blurring of vision after prolonged reading. He is an insomniac and is undergoing an acrimonious divorce with his wife.

He appears depressed, but well and there is no abnormal finding on general examination. The neurological signs are ill defined and variable. When first admitted, he appeared to have marked weakness in all four limbs. However, he does not appear to be producing maximal effort and when re-examined by the physician, he was found to have normal power in all four limbs when sufficiently encouraged. The tendon reflexes are barely obtainable in the arms and absent in both legs. Sensation is abnormal.

A. What is the diagnosis?
Ans: This patient has the Eaton-Lambert syndrome.

B. What other possibilities would you consider?
Ans: Myasthenia gravis and hyperthyroidism.

C. What investigation should be done?
Ans: Clinically, I would like to demonstrate that the strength of the patient increases with repetition. This may be demonstrated on EMG. A chest X-ray and CT scan should be performed.

Eaton-Lambert syndrome is associated with dysautonomic features and may include dryness of mouth and eyes, impotence, diminished sweating and orthostatic symptoms. The disorder afflicts men more often than women. The incidence of associated malignancy is 70% in man and 25% in women. In most cases of both sexes, the tumour is a small cell carcinoma of the lung.

It is considered to be an autoimmune disorder associated with diminished quantal release of acetylcholine. It is associated with other autoimmune disorders and appears to be HLA-linked (B8 and DRW 3 antigens). In the paraneoplastic Eaton-Lambert syndrome, evidence suggests there are antibodies directed against voltage-dependent calcium channels present both in the tumour and at distal motor nerve terminals.

Treatment is directed to the underlying neoplasm or autoimmune disease and towards augmentation of acetylcholine, with drugs that prolongs the pre-synaptic depolarisation, thereby enhancing calcium influx. Guanidine hydrochloride and 3–4 diaminopyridine may be beneficial either in autoimmune or the paraneoplastic Eaton-Lambert syndrome. Plasma exchange and immunosuppression may also be effective.

The diagnosis of Eaton-Lambert syndrome may signal the presence of a tumour long before it would otherwise be detected, permitting early removal. Treatment of the neuromuscular disorder involves plasma pheresis and immunosuppression.

It is interesting to know that both the syndrome of Eaton-Lambert and mysasthenia gravis have been demonstrated in animals by passive administration of botulin toxin, although the findings in botulism are variable and not all muscles are affected.

Q 059

A 31-year-old Persian teacher is admitted for weakness in her right arm and leg. This weakness is apparent when she walks, and her condition does not improve. Four days before she is admitted to the hospital, she had been seen in the casualty department for acute pain in the left upper abdomen. She was admitted for two days, but no cause was found and the symptoms resolved. She has had episodes of breathlessness usually related to exertion. She also complains of weight-loss, fever, episodic loss of vision. Her father had open-heart surgery at 30, but died on the table. She is a non-smoker and on contraceptive pills.

On examination, she has a very mild weakness of the face, arm and leg of the left side where the reflexes are brisker than the right with an extensor plantar response. Sensation is normal and she is in sinus rhythm with a heart rate of 90/min, blood pressure 110/80 mmHg. All arterial pulses are normal apart from those in the right foot which is absent. The house-officer documents a mid-diastolic murmur, but an opening snap is not audible. Investigation reveals mild normochromic normocytic anaemia, a high ESR of 90, and elevated serum Ig G concentration. Urea, creatinine and electrolytes are normal.

A. WHAT IS THE DIAGNOSIS?
ANS: This patient has left atrial myxoma.

Seven percent of cardiac myxoma are familial in nature, with an autosomal dominant transmission or part of a syndrome with complex abnormalities including lentiginous or pigmented naevi. There may also be primary nodular adrenal cortical disease with or without Cushing's syndrome, myxomatous mammary fibroadenomas, testicular tumours and pituitary adenomas with gigantism or acromegaly.

Certain constellations of findings have been referred to as the NAME syndrome (Naevi Atrial Myxoma, Myxoid neurofibroma and Ephelides) or the LAMB syndrome (Lentiginous, Atrial myxoma and Blue naevi).

An atrial myxoma may occur on the right or the left side. If it occurs in the right side, it may mimic the symptoms of tricuspid stenosis.

B. HOW WOULD YOU CONFIRM THE DIAGNOSIS?
ANS: 2-D echocardiography will readily diagnose a left atrial myxoma. This patient should also undergo a blood culture to rule out the possibility of infective endocarditis and be screened for systemic lupus erythromatosis.

Q 060

A 23-year-old actress develops numbness over the right side of the face with drooping of the face. By the time of admission several days later, she has also become weak and clumsy in her right arm and leg. She had noticed an occipital headache and feels nauseated and unsteady.

On examination, her vision and fundoscopy are normal. There is sustained nystagmus on gazing to the right and on looking ahead. She has sensory impairment of all modalities on the right side of her face, most marked over the upper lip and cheeks, but also extending over the forehead. The right side of the face is weak, also affecting eye closure. The tone and power are normal in the limbs, but there is incoordination of the right arm and leg. The tendon reflexes are brisk and both plantar reflexes are equivocal.

A. WHERE IS THE LESION?
ANS: In the cerebellum and the pons.

B. WHAT ARE THE POSSIBLE CAUSES OF THE CLINICAL PICTURE?
ANS: The possibilities are acoustic neuroma, multiple sclerosis and abscesses.

C. WHAT INVESTIGATION SHOULD BE DONE?
ANS: A CT scan or an MRI will show the lesions of multiple sclerosis.

Q 061

A 30-year-old Indian girl has been feeling unwell. She has been getting spontaneous contraction of the small muscles of the arms.

The investigations:
• Calcium – 1.74 mmol/L
• Phosphate – 1.52 mmol/L
• Albumin – 4 g/L
• Parathyroid hormones – 214 ng /L

A. WHAT IS THE MOST LIKELY DIAGNOSIS?
ANS: Pseudohypoparathyroidism. This is end-organ unresponsiveness to PTH. The patient may exhibit Chvostek and Trousseau's sign. This is also known as the Albright hereditary osteodystrophy. Pseudohypoparathyroidism is an inherited disorder characterised by end-organ resistance to PTH. The patient may also show partial resistance to other hormones that act by stimulation of the adenylcyclase, for example, PTH, vasopressin and glucagons.

Multiple exostosis may sometimes be seen in patients with pseudohypoparathyroidism. The metacarpals may be shortened in this condition and the patient may have a characteristic facies. This condition may be associated with mental retardation.

Q 062

Two and a half months after delivery, a lawyer suffers from fatigue, tachycardia and anxiety. She has been losing weight, and is feeling nervous and hot although the weather has not changed.

- Serum T_3 – 14 picomol/L.
- Free T_4 level – 47 picomol/L
- Serum TSH – less than 0.1 milliunits/L
- Thyroid isotopes scan – low uptake.
- Thyroid ultrasound – diffusely enlarged thyroid.

A. WHAT IS THE CAUSE OF THE SYMPTOMS?
ANS: This patient has postpartum thyroiditis.

The thyroid toxic phase may be followed in several months by a phase which is self limiting hypothyroidism. The hypothyroid component of this disease may be the only point at which it is diagnosed, as the hypothyroid period can be very brief.

There appears to be a wide geographical variation in the instance, approximately up to 8% of pregnant women may experience the symptoms postpartum. Postpartum thyroiditis may be associated with chronic thyroiditis with transient thyrotoxicosis (CT-TT). This syndrome has been designated as painless thyroiditis, silent thyroiditis, hyperthyroiditis, chronic thyroiditis with spontaneous resolving hyperthyroidism, or chronic thyroiditis with transient thyrotoxicosis. This implies the existence of hyperthyroidism is inappropriate since on-going production of thyroid hormones is negligible. Thyrotoxicosis in CT-TT may abate in 2–5 months.

Many patients have recurrent episodes of thyrotoxicosis of a similar nature, sometimes following pregnancy, in which case it is described as postpartum thyroiditis.

B. How would you differntiate CT/TT from Grave's disease?
Ans: This disorder can be differentiated from Grave's disease in the acute phase by the demonstration of absence of increase urinary iodine excretion. Definitive diagnosis of CT/TT can be made by thyroid biopsy.

Q 063

A 54-year-old vicar has had severe headache for six months and vomiting for four days. On examination, he is drowsy and appears pale, but not dehydrated. The blood pressure is 120/80 mmHg lying and 100/70 mmHg standing.

Investigation:
• Plasma sodium – 115 mmo1/L
• Potassium – 4.2 mmol/L
• Urea – 3.1 mmol/L
• Hb – 9 g/dl with normal indices

A. What is the most likely diagnosis?
Ans: Pituitary hypoadrenalism due to pituitary apoplexy. The potassium is under control of renin. The serum level of renin may be measured; this is reduced in apoplexy. One may peform an MRI or a CT scan to demonstrate the damaged pituitary.

B. What treatment should be given?
Ans: One should treat with cortisol (mineral corticosteroid) followed by thyroxine.

Q 064

A boxer is suspected to have acromegaly. Random growth hormone is elevated.
The following results were obtained after a 75 g glucose load.

Time (min)	Glucose level	Glucose Hormone level
0	4.5 mmol/L	26.4 milliunit/L
30	6.2 mmol/L	12.3 milliunit/L
60	8.7 mmol/L	8.9 milliunit/L
90	6.1 mmol/L	3 milliunit/L
120	5.7 mmol/L	1.2 milliunit/L
150	4.5 mmol/L	Less than 1 milliunit/L

A. What inference may be drawn from the results?
Ans: This patient does not have acromegaly.

Q 065

A 45-year-old Royal Air Force major is found on routine examination to have a blood pressure of 220/135 mmHg.

The biochemical results:
- Sodium – 144 mmol/L
- Potassium – 2.8 mmol/L
- Urea – 4.2 mmol/L
- Renin activity – 1.2 picomol/h/L
- Aldosterone – 78 picomols/L

A. What are your diagnoses?
Ans:
i) Congenital adrenal hyperplasia due to 11-betathydroxylase deficiency. In this condition, the cortisol and aldosterone levels will be low, and there will be a high degree of virilisation of the female. The dominant steroid, poorly excreted and deficient in 11-betahydroxylase congenital adrenal hyperplasia, is cortisone.
ii) Cushing's syndrome.
iii) Adrenal tumour
iv) Excessive liquorice intake. The ingestion of candy or chewing of tobacco containing certain forms of liquorice produces a syndrome similar to primary hyperaldosteronism. The sodium-retaining principle in such an agent is glycyrrhizimic acid which inhibits the 11-beta hydroxysteroid dehydrogenase, allowing cortisol to act as a mineral corticoid causing sodium retention, expansion of extra-

cellular fluid volume, and hypertension with a depressed plasma renin level and suppressed aldosterone level. This diagnosis is only made or excluded by careful study of the patient's medical history.

A 33-year-old paleontology student has had secondary amenorrhoea for the past five months. She has just return from a trip to Zimbabwe. She felt a sudden surge of warmth when she was doing research in the University library.

• The serum LH – 20 units/L (Normal levels – Follicle phase 3–12)
• The FSH – 36.4 units/L (Normal levels – Follicular phase 1–6)

A. WHAT IS THE DIAGNOSIS?
ANS: This patient has premature menopause. Premature ovarian failure or premature menopause occurs in women who cease menstruating prior to the age of 40. The ovaries are similar to the ovaries of post-menopausal women, namely, an absence of follicles as a result of accelerated follicular atresia. The premature ovarian failure may be due to ovarian antibodies.

This may be one of the components of polyglandular failure, together with adrenal insufficiency, hypothyroidism and other autoimmune disorders.

A rare form of ovarian failure is the resistant ovary syndrome in which the ovaries contain many follicles arrested in development prior to the antral state, possibly because of resistance to the action of FSH in the ovaries. This diagnosis would not be compatible with the lady's medical history as she has secondary amenorrhoea. Patients with resistant ovary syndrome may have primary amenorrhoea.

The predisposition to ischaemia heart disease is higher in women with premature menopause.

B. WHAT INVESTIGATION SHOULD BE PERFORMED?
ANS: The estradiol level should be measured. One should attempt to detect antibodies against the ovarian tissues. Chromosomal analysis should be performed for Turner's syndrome (which may be present as mosaicism. The most common form of mosaicism is 45 XO/ 46 XX).

MRI of the pituitary fossa should be done. The TSH level should be performed to rule out hypothyroidism.

Q 067

A 22-year-old chef has a 9-month history of amenorrhoea. Her menarche was at the age of 15. The periods have always been infrequent and she is worried it might be due to the condiments she is using for her cooking as she is learning to make exotic sauces.

On examination, no abnormality was found.

- Prolactin level – 650 MU/L (increased)
- LH – 22 units/L
- FSH – 6 units/L
- Estradiol – 300 picomols/L
- Thyroid function test – normal

A. WHAT IS THE DIAGNOSIS?

ANS: This lady has PCOD (Polycytis Ovarian disease).

This is a condition with chronic anovulation with oestrogen present. Women with chronic anovulation who experience withdrawal bleeding after administration of progesterone are said to be in a state of estrus due to acyclic production of oestrogen. This is usually oestrone by extraglandular aromatisation of circulating androstenedione.

The women are usually hirsute, obese and may complain of amenorrhoea or ologomenorrhoea. When spontaneous uterine bleeding occurs in subjects with PCOD, it is unpredictable with respect to duration and amount. On occasion, the bleeding may be severe. The dysfunctional uterine bleeding is usually due to oestrogen breaking through. This disorder may be transmitted as an autosomal dominant or an X-link trait and was originally described by Stein as characterised by enlarged polycystic ovaries, but the syndrome and its accompanying endocrine abnormalities are now known to be associated with a variety of pathological findings in the ovaries. Some may result in the enlargement of the ovaries and none of which are diagnostic.

The common finding is a white smooth sclerotic ovary with a thickening capsule, multiple follicle cysts in various stages of atresia, a hyperplastic theca and stroma and rare or absent corpura albicans.

B. How would you treat this woman?

Ans: The aim is to interrupt the self-perpetuating cycle by decreasing ovarian androgen secretion (with resection or oral contraceptive agents), decreasing peripheral oestrogen formation (weight reduction) and enhancing FSH secretion (administration of clomiphene, human menopausal gonadotropin (hMG), LHRH (gonadorelin) by portable infusion pump or purified FSH (Urofollitropin).)

The choice of therapy depends on the clinical findings and the needs of the patient. Weight reduction is necessary in those who are obese. If the woman is not hirsute and does not desire pregnancy, periodic withdrawal menses can be induced by prescribing medroxyprogesterone acetate 10 days/month. Such treatment prevents the development of endometrial hyperplasia. If the woman is hirsute, but does not desire pregnancy, the ovarian and, possibly, the adrenal component of the androgen production can be suppressed with combined oestrogen-progesterone or oral contraceptive agents.

Combined oral contraceptives are also indicated if prolonged and excessive menstrual bleeding is experienced. Once androgen excess is controlled, treatment of hair growth by shaving or eletrolysis may be indicated.

C. This lady desires to be pregnant. Is there any means of achieving this?

Ans: Induction of ovulation is necessary. Administer Clomiphene, which promotes ovulation in three-quarters of cases of treatment with hMG, urofollitropin or gonadorelin. Pre-treatment with LHRH analogues prior to hMG urofollitropin or gonadorelin can improve the ovulation and pregnancy rate.

A wedge resection of the ovary is rarely indicated because of the development of adhesion, but it may sometimes be successful.

Q 068

A 53-year-old attorney has a 6-month history of dysphagia, dyspnoea, fatigue, ankle swelling, and has also been experiencing a tingling sensation in his legs, and visual difficulties that make his appearance in court problematic. He smokes cigars and has no other significant history. He appears ill and breathless on minimal exertion and complains of cold extremities.

The patient has telangiectasia over the right side of his chin. His blood pressure is 180/120 mmHg and his JVP is elevated at 7.2 cm. His heart sounds are soft, but normal. There are bilateral basal crackles, the liver is enlarged by four finger-breadths. There is gross peripheral oedema, but all peripheral pulses are preserved.

Investigations:
- Hb – 13 g/dL
- WBC – 9.5 x 10^9 /L
- ESR – 2 mm/h
- Urea – 13 mmol/L
- Creatinine – 150 µmol/L
- Bilirubin – 26 mmol/L
- ALT – 252 IU/L
- ECG sinus rhythm – right bundle branch block, with left anterior hemiblock and T-wave inversion in leds I, AVL and AVR.
- Chest X-ray – global cardiomegaly with mottled shadowing in the mid and lower zone.
- Peripheral smear – hypersegmented neutrophils.

A. WHAT IS THE DIAGNOSIS?

ANS: This patient has scleroderma with cardiomyopathy, attributable to myocardial fibrosis.

Radioisotope studies show left ventricular function abnormality compatible to myocardial fibrosis. The characteristic pathological band necrosis results from cardiac muscle damage caused by intermittent vasoconstriction of coronary vessels. Patients may experience angina pectoris even though coronary angiograms are normal. He has hypertension secondary to renal involvement of scleroderma. Renal failure is the leading cause of death in scleroderma accounting for almost 50% of death.

Angiographic studies of patients with scleroderma show constriction of the intralobular arteries, a stimulate vasospasm of digital arteries seen in Raynaud's phenomenon. The renal vascular involvement in scleroderma is characterised by a demonstration of small arteries undergoing intimal proliferation, medial thinning and increased collagen within the adventitial layer. Fibroid changes in the wall of the afferent arterioles and microinfarcts may occur. Tubules are often atrophic.

Aggressive control of systemic arterial pressure is critical in the therapy of scleroderma and may limit renal injury by blunting the process of nephrosclerosis. In a scleroderma or renal crisis, prompt treatment with beta blockers, minoxidil and angiotensin-1 converting enzyme may reverse acute renal failure. ACE inhibitors have changed the prognosis of scleroderma.

Bilateral basal crackles in the lungs suggest fibrosing alveolitis, associated with scleroderma. In scleroderma, the dilated blood vessels have a unique configuration and are known as mat telangiectasia. The lesions are broad macules that usually measure 2–7 mm in diameter. The common locations for mat telangiectasia are the face, oral mucosa and hands, as well as other peripheral sites that are prone to intermittent ischaemia.

Periungual telangiectasia is pathogonomic of the three major connective tissue diseases - SLE, scleroderma and dermatomyositis. They occur in 30% of these patients. In scleroderma and dermatomyositis, there is a loss of capillary loops and those which remain are markedly dilated.

B. What is the pathology behind the neurological signs described by this patient?

Ans: This patient has B12 deficiency due to reduced intestinal motility and jejunal pseudodiverticulosis and leading to stasis of intestinal contents and bacterial overgrowth.

The bacteria consumes vitamin B12 and the synthesis of folic acid is the rent the bacteria pay for inhabiting the bowel. The serum B12 will, therefore, be low and the folate level elevated. Therapy with somastatin analogue octreotide has stimulated intestinal motility, reduced bacterial overgrowth and ameliorated obstructive gut symptoms.

Q 069

A 46-year-old zoologist has a 3-month history of weight-loss with profuse diarrheoa, including the three days before hospitalisation for her annual check-up.

Examination, including sigmoidoscopy, is normal apart from reduced skin turgor. She appears thin.

- Hb – 13.2 g/dl
- WBC – 8.0 x10⁹/l
- ESR – 2.3 mm/h
- Urea – 16 mmo/l
- Sodium – 131 mmol/l
- Potassium – 3.2 mmol/l
- Bicarbonate – 24 mmol/l
- LFT, gamma-globulins. Thyroid function, stool culture and microscopy, jejunal biopsy and barium studies – normal
- 24-hour fecal fat – 18 mmols and weight 1,200 g

A. What is the initial therapy?
Ans: It is imperative to correct the electrolyte imbalance immediately. One should not correct the sodium deficit abruptly as this may lead to cerebellopontine myelinolysis (CPM). It is for this reason hypertonic saline should not be used for the correction of hyponatriemia.

B. What investigation would aid in reaching the diagnosis?
Ans: Gut hormone profile and colonoscopy.

C. What is the most likely diagnosis?
Ans: This patient has secretory diarrhoea. The clinical picture in this lady is highly suggestive of lipoma. This may be associated with the watery diarrhoea hypokalemia achlorhydria syndrome (WDHA).

This is characterised by massive secretory diarrhoea, achlorhydria, hypokalemia, hypomagnesemia, hypercalcemia without hyperparathyroidism, and in some cases flushing, myopathy or nephropathy.

However, not all patients with WDHA have a lipoma. In such cases, alternative mediators of intestinal secretion have been postulated.

D. What are the other causes of diarrhoea?
Ans: The other causes of secretory diarrhoea are cholera, laxative abuse, carcinoid syndrome, inflammatory bowel syndrome, Zollinger-Ellison syndrome, HIV and collagen disorder involving the gut or microscopic colitis.

Q 070

A 76-year-old cartographer has had pale mushy stools for seven months. She improved temporarily for the last six weeks after recovering from flu. Several years ago, she had surgery for a ruptured duodenal ulcer.

Physical examination is normal and sigmoidoscopy does not demonstrate any abnormality. The stools are steatorrhoeic.

Investigation:
- Hb – 10 g/d1
- ESR – 3 mm/h
- Serum B12 – 50 mmol/l
- Serum folate – normal
- Albumin – 33 g/l
- Calcium – 2.1 mmol/l
- Phosphate – 0.7 mmol/l

A. WHAT IS THE DIAGNOSIS?

ANS: This patient has the blind loop secondary to bacterial colonisation following gastrectomy.

The diagnosis may be confirmed by Schilling's test. Bacterial overgrowth may be detected by aspirating fluid from the upper small intestine through an endoscope or a small intestinal tube placed under fluoroscope guidance and finding a bacterial colony count greater than 10^5 mm.

The diagnosis of bacterial overgrowth may also be suggested by an increase in exhaled $^{14}CO_2$ within 60 minutes of ingestion of lg of 14C-D-Xylose (14C- Xylose breath test) or after ingestion of 14-Cholyglycine (bile acid breadth test) or the detection of the increased breathing of H_2 within the first two hours after the ingestion of either glucose or rice-flour (breath hydrogen test).

This patient should be treated with antibiotics; the response to antibiotics is supportive of this diagnosis. One may perform the Schilling's test part 3 (after giving antibiotics).

Q 071

A 23-year-old lecturer of comparative religion has had a sudden onset of severe upper abdominal pain and vomiting. He was admitted to the hospital with a similar episode two years ago.

Examination shows marked epigastric tenderness, guarding and absent bowel sounds. He admits to drinking heavily and appears pale with clammy hands. Pulse is 100/min and BP 110/70 mmHg.

Investigation:
- Hb – 12.5 g/dl
- WBC – 19 x 10⁹/L
- Serum amylase – 3,700 U/dl
- ECG and CXR – normal

He is treated in the ICU and appeared to recover within the next few days. His serum amylase three weeks later is 900.

A. WHAT IS THE DIAGNOSIS?
ANS: This patient has developed pancreatic pseudocyst following the episode of acute pancreatitis. This occurs in 15% of patients.

Pseudocysts do not have epithelial lining and the walls consist of neurotic, granulation and fibrous tissue. Pseudocyst is preceeded by pancreatitis in 90% of cases and by trauma in 10%. Most of the cases are located in the body or tail of the pancreas and 10% in the head of the pancreas. Some patients have two or more pseudocysts. A palpable tender mass may be found in the left upper abdomen and the diagnosis is readily confirmed by USG.

B. NAME SOME CONDITIONS IN WHICH THE ACUTE CONDITIONS ARE ASSOCIATED WITH NORMAL SERUM AMYLASE DESPITE PANCREATIC DESTRUCTION.
ANS:
i) Hyperlipdaemia type 4 which interferes with the amylase assay.
ii) A late assay and the acute onset of chronic recurrent pancreatitis where there is inadequate pancreatic mass to produce sufficient amylase.

C. SEVERAL DAYS LATER, THE PATIENT BECAME HYPOTENSIVE. ON AUSCULTATION THERE WAS A LOCALISED BRUIT OVER THE MASS. THE BLOOD TEST SHOWS A SUDDEN DROP IN HAEMOGLOBIN AND HAEMATOCRIT LEVELS AND THE STOOLS ARE NEGATIVE FOR OCCULT BLOOD. WHAT HAS HAPPENED?

Ans: This patient has haemorrhage from a pseudocyst. The patient should be operated on immediately.

If this patient's pseudocyst is stable and uncomplicated and the ultrasound study shows a decrease in size, conservative treatment is indicated. Conversely, patients with a pseudocyst which is expanding and complicated by rupture, haemorrhage or an abscess, should be operated on.

Using ultrasound or CT guidance, a sterile chronic pseudocyst can be treated safely with single or repeated needle aspiration or with cathether drainage. A success rate of 50–75% can be achieved. The success rate with an infected pseudocyst is considerably less, 40–50%. Patients not responding to drainage require surgery.

Pseudoaneurysms develop in up to 10% of patients with acute pancreatitis in sites reflecting the distribution of pseudocyst and fluid collection. This diagnosis should be suspected in patients with pancreatitis who develop either a upper gastrointestinal bleed without an obvious cause or in whom a contrast enhanced lesion is within or adjacent to a suspected pseudocyst, as determined by a high resolution CT examination. Arteriography is necessary to confirm the diagnosis.

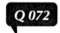

Q 072

A 15-year-old X-ray technician's apprentice has acute right loin pain, but apart from being relatively short for his age, has no other abnormalities on physical examination. An abdominal x-ray reveals a bilateral, multiple spots of opacity in both renal areas.

Investigations:
- Sodium – 138 mmol/l
- Potassium – 2.6 mmol/l
- Urea – 7 mmol/l
- Creatinine – 111 μmol/l
- Chloride – 119 mmol/l
- Bicarbonate – 22 mmol/l
- Urine pH – 7
- Trace proteins – +
- Blood – ++
- Culture – sterile

A. WHAT IS THE DIAGNOSIS?

ANS: This patient has nephrocalcinosis secondary to distal renal tubular acidosis. This is also called Type I renal tubular acidosis, associated with hypercalcuria, osteomalacia, nephrocalcinosis and lithiasis.

The acidosis should be corrected as completely as possible in patients with Type I RTA as this will avoid hypercalcuria and osteomalacia. The renal tubular acidosis type I is characterised by the inability to lower the urine pH normally. There is a reduced acid excretion. It is inherited in an autosomal dominant mode and may be associated with periodic paralysis, hypokalemia, non-anion gap metabolic acidosis, growth retardation and rickets.

Q 073

A 42-year-old actor is suffering from fever, malaise and generalised aches and pains. Three weeks after the onset of his condition, later he notes a discharge from the right ear and some hoarseness of speech. Treatment with cephalosporins and nasal spray relieves his symptoms. One week later he notices the painful swelling of his right knee and right elbow, followed by a transient erythematous skin rash.

On examination, he has ankle oedema and +++ proteinuria from the Dipstick test. There is a family history of tuberculosis (mother) and late onset hypertension. He does not smoke, but drinks social amounts of alcohol. He had exophthalmos and lateral conjunctivitis. His temperature is 38°C. Otoscopy reveals serous otitis media in the left ear and the mucous membrane of the nose is swollen and crusted. An erythematous papular rash is present over the trunk and right arm. His blood pressure is 195/90 mmHg. Pedal oedema is present. A 3-finger nontender hepatomegaly is palpated, but he is not clinically jaundiced. The chest is clear. A CXR shows poorly defined rounded soft shadows in both lung-fields, and small left pleural effusion.

Results of investigations:
- Hb – 11.2 g/dl
- WBC – 7.3 x 10^9/L
- Platelets – 700 x 10^9/L
- ESR – 80 mm/h
- Urine blood – ++
- Urine protein – +++

- Urea – 12
- Creatinine – 172 µmol/l
- Sodium –141 mmol/l
- Potassium – 4.9 mmol/l
- Bicarbonate – 28 mmol/l

A. WHAT IS THE MOST LIKELY DIAGNOSIS?

ANS: This patient has Wegener's granulomatosis.

This is a distinct pathological entity characterised by granulomatous vasculitis of the upper and lower respiratory tracts, together with glomerulonephritis. In addition, a variable degree of disseminated vasculitis involving both small arteries and veins may occur. This is rare in blacks and the male-to-female ratio is 1:1. The disease rarely occurs before adolescence and the mean age of onset is 40 years.

This disease is characterised by antineutrophil cytoplasmic antibodies called c-ANCA (c-ANCA refers to the coarse granular pattern observed by immunofluorescence microscopy when serum antibodies bind to cytoplasmic components on indicator neutrophils). C-ANCA is a sensitive (88%) and specific (95%) marker for Wegener's granulomatosis. Renal biopsy will confirm the diagnosis of glomerulonephritis.

Lymphomaoid granulomatosis has to be differentiated from Wegner's. This condition is characterised by lung, skin, central nervous system and kidney involvement in which atypical lymphoctoid and plasmacytoid cells infiltrate tissue in an angioinvasive manner. In this regard, it clearly differs from Wegener's granulomatosis in that it is not an inflammatory vasculitis in the classical sense but an infiltration of vessels with atypical mononuclear cells and granulomas in involved tissues.

Approximately 50% of patients develop true malignant lymphoma. The presence of c-ANCA is extremely helpful in the differentiation from all the preceding diseases.

B. HOW WOULD YOU TREAT THESE PATIENTS?

ANS: Wegener's granulomatosis is regarded as fatal within a few months after the onset of clinically overt renal disease. Glucocorticoids alone led to some symptomic improvement. It has been well established that the treatment of choice of this disease is cyclophosphamide. The leucocyte count should be monitored during therapy and the dose should be adjusted to maintain the count above 3,000/mm3, which generally maintains a neutrophil count approximately 1,500/microL. Clinical remission can be induced in this manner and maintained without causing severe leucopenia with its associated risk of infection. Cyclophosphamide should be continued for one year following the induction of complete remission, and tapered and discontinued thereafter.

With this regime, the prognosis is excellent with marked improvement seen in 90% of patients and complete remission in 75% of patients. A number of patients who develop irreversible renal failure but who achieve remission on appropriate therapy, have undergone successful renal transplantation. If the patients cannot tolerate cyclophosphamide, azathioprine should be used. Reports have indicated that trimethoprim sulphamethoxazole may be of benefit in the treatment of Wegener's granulomatosis, but there is no firm data to substantiate this in patients with serious renal and pulmonary disease. A regiment of methotrexate, up to 25 mg/week with glucocorticoid on alternate days, has shown some promise in treatment of patients with moderate disease.

Q 074

A 23-year-old film director was returning from a movie set when he was mugged by two youths who chased him for several blocks. He had to climb over a wall to get away from them. The following day he noticed pain and stiffness, especially in the pectoral muscles where he had been hit. He then passed a small volume of dark coloured urine. The patient is a member of Alcoholics Anonymous and has been attempting to quit smoking.

On examination, there is redness and swelling with tenderness of the pectoral muscles and his back. The blood pressure is 160/180 mmHg and the rest of the physical examination is normal.

Investigations:
- Hb – 13.5 g/dl
- WBC – 8.4 x 10⁹/L
- Platelets – 164 x 10⁹/L
- Urea – 24 mmol/L
- Creatinine – 790 mmol/L
- Sodium – 130 mmol/L
- Potassium – 6.7 mmol/L

- Bicarbonate – 18 mmol/L
- Calcium – 1.8 mmol/L
- Phosphate – 2.9 mmol/L
- Bilirubin – 25 miromol/L
- Alkaline phosphatase – 195 IU/L
- SGOT – 92 IU/L
- Total protein – 61 g/L
- Albumin – 29 g/L
- Uric acid – 1.4 mmol/L
- Urine dipstick test – ++ for blood and + for protein

A. WHAT IS THE DIAGNOSIS?

ANS: This patient has rhabdomyolysis with myoglobinuria. The myoglobin and the urates are toxic and may block the tubules. This leads to renal failure.

Studies in Israel, based on crush injuries suggest that immediate intravenous alkalinisation of the patient will reduce the probability of renal failure. Should the urine alkalinisation be initiated early, the prognosis for renal failure is very good.

Hypercalcaemia may be noted as the muscles recover. Mild hypercalcaemia during recovery may be a consequence of transient hyperparathyroidism or due to mobilisation of sequested calcium from injured muscle.

B. IS THE CONSUMPTION OF ALCOHOL RELATED TO THIS CONDITION IN ANY WAY?

ANS: Rhabdomyolysis occurs in chronic alcoholics who have become acutely hypophosphataemic during the course of alcohol withdrawal. Hypophosphataemia rhabdomyolysis also occurs, rarely, during treatment of diabetic ketoacidosis with hyperalimentation, or while feeding malnourished patients. In alcoholics, evidence of muscle cell injury preceeds the occurrence of hyperphosphataemia.

Presumably, severe hypophosphataemia triggers the induction of rhabdomyolysis. This syndrome can be reproduced experimentally. It does not occur if hypophosphataemia is prevented during hyperalimentation. This is obviously not the reason for the patient's rhabdomyolysis as described.

Q 075

A 68-year-old wife of an immigration director visits her physician complaining of tiredness. He finds her to have a haemoglobin of 8.3 g/dl and gives her a 3-month course of iron. There is no improvement. She is then referred to the outpatient department.

On examination, she appears generally fit but pale. Her blood pressure is 183/94 mmHg. There is ankle oedema.

Investigation:
- Hb – 8.3 g/dl
- WBC – 5.7 x 10^9/L
- Platelets – 90 x 10^9/L
- Urea – 36.4 mmol/L
- Creatinine – 690 mmol/L
- Sodium – 131 mmol/L
- Potassium – 4.8 mmol/L
- Bicarbonate – 23 mmol/L
- Total protein – 84 g/L
- Albumin – 36 g/L
- Calcium – 3 mmol/L
- Phosphate – 1.8 mmol/L
- Bilirubin – 14 µmol/L
- SGOT – 26 IU/L
- Alkaline phosphatase – 124 IU/L
- Glucose – 4.6 mmol/L
- Uric asid – 0.93 mmol/L
- Urine analysis – protein-trace

A. WHAT IS THE MOST LIKELY DIAGNOSIS?
ANS: This patient has multiple myeloma.

Her renal function should be protected by dialysis. She should be treated with allopurinol to prevent gout, cyclophosphamide and steroids (for hypercalcaemia). The calcium level should be lowered with rehydration and a combination of loop diuretics. The calcium level can also be reduced by the use of mithramycin. The classic triad of myeloma is marrow plasmacytosis, more than 10% lytic bone lesion and/or urine M component.

Myeloma increases with age. Patients with myeloma are susceptible to bacterial infections. The most common infections are pneumonia and pyelonephritis and the most common pathogens are streptococcus pneumonea, staphylococcus aureus, klebsiella pneumonia, E. coli and other gram negative organisms in the urinary tract. Renal failure occurs in one quarter of patients with myeloma. Hypercalcaemia is the most common cause of renal failure. Glomerular deposits of amyloid, hyperuricaemia, recurrent infections and occasional infiltration of the kidneys by myeloma cells, all may contribute to renal dysfunction. Tubular damage associated with the excretion of light chains is almost always present. Normally, light chains are filtered, reabsorbed in the tubules and catabolised. With the increase in the amount of light chains to the tubules, the tubular cells become overloaded with this protein and tubular damage results, either directly from light chain toxic effects or from the release of intracellular lysosomal enzymes.

The earliest manifestation of this tubular damage is the Adult Fanconi syndrome (type II proximal tubular acidosis) with increased loss of glucose, amino acids and defect of the ability of the kidney to acidify and concentrate the urine. Proteinuria is not accompanied by hypertension and the protein is almost all light chains. Patients with myeloma have a decreased anion gap because the M component is cationic, resulting in retention of chloride. This is often accompanied by pseudohyponatraemia because each volume of serum has less water as a result of increased protein.

Q 076

A 22-year-old pilot, who is working in an aircraft carrier, has nodes on the right side of his neck. This was noticed by his wife when they were intimate. He is otherwise well and has no significant history.

On examination, he has four very firm nodes measuring 2 cm on the right side of his neck. He has no other lymphadenopathy, no hepatosplenomegaly and no mass palpable in the abdomen. Rectal examination is normal. The lymph nodes are biopsied and the histological report showed that it is compatible with adenocarcinoma.

A. WHAT OTHER CLINICAL EXAMINATION WOULD YOU UNDERTAKE?
ANS: I would perform a testicular examination.

B. WHAT PRIMARY SITE FOR THIS CANCER WOULD YOU CONSIDER MOST LIKELY?
ANS: The gut, the testes (teratoma), the thyroid and the lungs.

C. WHAT FURTHER DIAGNOSTIC TEST WOULD YOU RECOMMEND?
ANS: HCG, alpha fetoprotein and an ultrasound of the testes.

Q 077

A 38-year-old Indian missile scientist had a routine blood count performed. Six years earlier he had a severe cerebral vascular accident, but is otherwise well. The following blood results were obtained:

Results:
- Hb – 15.8 g/dl
- MCV – 71 fl (normal 80–100)
- Red cell count – 6.5 x 10^{12}/L
- MCH – 25 pg (normal 27–32)
- MCHC – 33.1 g/dl (normal 32–36)
- WBC – 6.5 x 10^9/L
- Platelets – 215 x 10^9/L

A. WHAT ARE THE POSSIBLE DIAGNOSES?
ANS: One should consider the possibilities of
i)   Thalassaemia with Gasboik syndrome (stress polycythaemia – It is a relative polycythaemia seen in professionals and executives who are inactive.)
ii) Polycythemia with iron deficiency anaemia.

Q 078

A 57-year-old principal of a nursing school has shortness of breath which has worsened over the last few weeks. She finds it difficult to climb the stairs in the hospital in which she works, as the lift sometimes does not function. She does not have a history of bleeding and haemoptysis. She appears pale and has raised JVP. Apart from bilateral ankle oedema, there is no other finding.

Investigation:
- Hb – 4 g/dl
- WBC – 8.5 x 10⁹/L with normal differential count;
- Platelets – 303 x 10⁹/L
- Reticulocytes – 0.2%
- The blood film showed normochromic normocytic anaemia.
- Chest X-ray showed Kerley B lines, upper lobe diversion and pulmonary oedema. There is also a large shadow in the mediastinum area.
- Urea – 5.5 mmol/L
- Albumin – 41 g/L
- Total protein – 54 g/L

A. WHAT IS THE DIAGNOSIS AND WHY IS THE PROTEIN LEVEL LOW?
ANS: This patient has thymoma with red cell aplasia and hypogammaglobulimaemia.

This is a rare acquired form of pure red cell aplasia. About one-third of the patients have thymoma. There is also an association between thymoma and myasthenia gravis. However, this is not suggested in the case history elicited. The protein is low due to the presence of hypogammaglobulinaemia. Erythropoiesis is inhibited by a complement fixing Ig G immunoglobulin which has selective cytotoxic effects on the marrow erythroblasts. A smaller number of patients have been noted to have an inhibitor against erythropoietin.

B. WHAT OTHER CONDITIONS MAY BE ASSOCIATED WITH THIS HAEMATOLOGICAL DYSFUNCTION?
ANS: Pure red cell aplasia may be associated with hypogammaglobulinaemia (as in this case), SLE, T-gamma lymphocytosis and AIDS.

Occasionally, pure red cell aplasia is encountered in T-cell chronic lymphatic leukaemia. The circulating T-cells in this condition are distinguished by the presence of receptors for the Fc portion of Ig G.

C. HOW WOULD YOU MANAGE THIS PATIENT?
ANS: These patients are totally dependant on red blood cell transfusion.

A thymectomy may induce a remission in 50% of patients. If the thymus is normal, the thymectomy is of no benefit. Patients without thymonia or those with unsuccessful thymectomy should receive glucocorticoids in combination with immunosuppressive agents such as cyclophosphamide, azathioprine, cyclosporins and anti-thymocyte globulin. Treatment often results in prolonged remission and disappearance of the inhibitor.

Q 079

A 25-year-old assistant of a 5-star hotel suffers a massive deep vein thrombosis (DVT) six days postpartum. She had a previous episode of DVT when she was on the pill. She was treated with intravenous heparin for five days with excellent control. Warfarin was stopped. She is due to be discharged, but the deep vein thrombosis worsens. She cries in pain. It is feared her limbs are at risk. The skin of the leg affected by the DVT has undergone necrosis.

A. HOW WOULD MANAGE THIS PATIENT?

ANS: The author has performed emergency femoral surgical embolectomy for a similar problem after angiography has delineated the extent of the pathology.

I would look for the antithrombin III, protein C and protein S deficiency and the lupus anticoagulant. Antithrombin III, protein C, protein S and the tissue factor pathway inhibitor (TFPI) are the most important inhibitors that collectively maintain the blood in its fluid form. The correlation between the protein C and protein S levels and the risk of thrombosis are not as precise as that of antithrombin III. Asymptomatic individuals with protein C deficiency have been discovered. This observation raises the possibility that a yet undiscovered comorbid condition is present in symptomatic patients.

Since only a fraction of the available protein S is bound to the C4b-binding proteins and is unavailable for coagulation reactions, it may be important to measure the free and total protein S or to have a concomitant measurement of C4b-binding protein for maximum accuracy. When patients with protein C and protein S deficiency are put on warfarin, this vitamin K antagonist, which lower the levels of procoagulant factor II, VII, IX and X, may reduce the concentration of protein C and protein S sufficiently to nullify the desired antithrombotic effect. In fact, it may result in a procoagulant state. Patients with homozygous protein C deficiency require periodic plasma infusion rather than oral anti-coagulant to prevent recurrent intravascular coagulation and thrombosis.

Deficiency of protein C and protein S are usually autosomal dominant disorders and the deficiency in the two proteins causes an identical syndrome of recurrent venous thrombosis and pulmonary embolism. In addition, rare patients with homozygous protein C deficiency have fulminant neonatal intravascular coagulation and require prompt diagnosis and treatment. Hence the baby should also be assayed for the protein C and protein S levels if the mother is diagnosed to be deficient.

A 34-year-old man shows up at the hospital complaining of severe epigastric discomfort, but it does not radiate to the back or the upper quadrants. He says he had a peptic ulcer which required an emergency operation.

On examination he is afebrile, with marked tenderness in the epigastric region, but no abdominal guarding, no rebound tenderness, and the bowel sounds are normal. His abdomen looks like a battle field with many previous operations. Fibreoptic gastroscopy shows a bleeding ulcer crater. No free gas can be seen on the chest X-ray and the surgeon considered an emergency laparotomy. The patient then claims he has haemophilia. He does not have any record and had lost his hospital identification card. The staff positioned was part of a skeletal crew as this was 3 am in a small district hospital without any sophisticated laboratory support. This patient was referred from the prison with a complaint of severe abdominal pain. There are many contradictions and inconsistencies in the history that the patient gives.

His bleeding time, as well as the PT, is found to be prolonged. The full blood count is normal.

A. WHAT IS THE DIAGNOSIS?

ANS: This prisoner is psychologically disturbed and may have surreptitiously ingested coumarin and aspirin, causing a bleeding peptic ulcer and a prolonged PT. The plasma coumarin level can be measured to confirm such ingestion. The bleeding time is prolonged as he is also taking aspirin and this can be confirmed by an aspirin level measurement.

This patient is suffering from Munchausen's syndrome and should be evaluated by a consultant psychiatrist. This syndrome was named after Baron von Munchausen for his inventive lying of bizarre adventures.

A full blood count should be performed and the partial thromboplastin time should be done. The gastric ulcer should be treated by an endoscopic cauterisation with a heater probe or clips. The tip of the endoscopic probe may be used to cauterise the bleeding vessels and prevent bleeding. This patient should receive intravenous ranitidine. To correct the prolongation of the bleeding time associated with aspirin, fresh platelet transfusion may be required. Aspirin contributes to the development of gastric ulcers by interruption to the gastric mucosal barrier, permitting back diffusion of hydrogen ions which may injure gastric mucosa. They reduce gastric mucosal secretion and gastric and duodenal bicarbonate secretion and increase gastric acid secretion. Depletion of mucosal prostaglandin impairs gastric epithelial cell reconstitution after injury.

This patient may be treated with fresh frozen plasma (FFP) and cryoprecipitates. These are the major plasma components used for patients with clotting disorder. FFP contains all coagulation factors found in fresh plasma. Each 250ml unit infusion raises most coagulation factors' levels 3–5%. FFP is used for bleeding patients with multiple coagulation factor deficiency, such as that may occur in severe liver disease and dilutional coagulopathy. Warfarin induced deficiency of vitamin K dependant factors may be rapidly reversed by FFP. But ordinarily, vitamin K administration induces a smooth reversal in 6–12 hours. FFP is rarely indicated for prolongation of prothrombin time less than 1.5 times normal.

Cryoprecipitate contains about half the factor VIII activity of fresh frozen plasma in one-tenth of the volume, is simple to prepare and is produced in hospital blood-banks. It must be stored frozen, and thawed and pooled before administration. Most patients utilise partially purified factor VIII concentrate, which is prepared from multiple donors and supplied lyophilized powder. It can be refrigerated and reconstituted just prior to use. Factor VIII therapy has increased in safety. Heating of lyophilized factor VIII under carefully controlled conditions can inactivate HIV without destroying factor VIII coagulant activity. Highly purified factor VIII can be produced, absorbing and eluding factor VIII from monoclonal antibody columns. Recombinant factor VIII has just completed clinical trials and is now being marketed.

The role of fresh whole blood is poorly defined and is rarely advantageous. During refrigerated storage, whole blood affinity increases as red cell 2–3 DPG falls. Other changes include a rise in extra-cellular potassium and lactate concentration and a decline in pH. Blood less than 24 hours old may benefit children undergoing cardiopulmonary bypass. It is sad that thousands of haemophiliacs were infected with HIV by receiving HIV infected fresh frozen plasma or concentrates of clotting factors. Approximately 2,000 have developed AIDS. One study estimates the risk of HIV I infection via transfused blood from a HIV infected but seronegative donor, ranges from one in 40,000 to one in 250,000, while in another study it was estimated 1:61,000.

Q 081

A 63-year-old lady, married to a carpenter who specialises in imitation Victorian furniture, has a painless rash over the shin. This developed during the last six weeks. She has just returned from Spain where the physician diagnosed contact dermatitis and prescribed topical steroids, but her condition did not improve. She gives a 5-month history of lethargy, aching joints and experiencing Raynaud's phenomenon. She also has parasthesia and loss of sensation in the right lower limb in the area supply of the lateral popliteal nerve. She has a right ulnar neuropathy and sensory loss of the right lower limb in the stoking distribution. She is an occasional social drinker and has extensive palpable purpuric rash over the shin with areas of ulceration. Her fingers are cold with poor capillary filling, but all the peripheral pulses are present. She has a painless palpable liver and spleen.

Investigation:
- Hb – 11.1 g/dL
- WBC – 6 x 10⁹/L
- Platelets – 243 x 10⁹/L
- Sodium – 135 mmol/L
- Potassium – 4.3 mmol/L
- Urea – 8.9 mmol/L
- Creatinine – 149 µmols/L
- Albumin – 32 g/L
- Total proteins – 83 g/L
- Calcium – 2.4 mmol/L

- AST – 75 IU/L
- ALT – 67 IU/L
- IU/L Gamma glutamyl transferase – 39 IU/L
- Urine protein – ++
- Urine blood – trace
- Microscopy – inactive sediment
- Rh factor – 1–8
- DNA binding – 1%
- C_2 – 33%
- C_3 – 68%
- C_4 – 27%
- Skin biopsy – leucocytoplastic vasculitis

A. WHAT IS THE DIAGNOSIS?

ANS: This patient has essential mixed cryoglobulinaemia (usually Ig G and Anti Ig G).

Essential cryoglobulinaemia was initially reported to be associated with hepatitis B. Patients with this syndrome usually have chronic liver disease, but the association with HBV infection is controversial. Recent re-evaluation in patients with EMC suggests instead that a substantial portion have chronic HCV infection. The circulating immune complex of EMC contain HCV RNA in a concentration that exceeds its serum concentration. This observation argues against secondary trapping of HCV in the immune complexes and favours a primary role for the virus for the pathogenesis of EMC. Following the EMC, hepatitis B, occult fungal and bacterial infection may be found to underly this syndrome.

Circulating cryoimmunoglobulins are also found in chronic infections and probably represent circulating immune complexes with unusual physical properties. Serum complement, particularly the C_4 component, are depressed. This may be associated with athralgia, increased weakness and unexplained nephirits.

Plasmapheresis will temporarily lower the level of globulins, remove immune complexes and improve this patient's condition. Long-term management must include control of the underlying disease which produces the abnormal globulin or immune complex. The cutaneous lesions are excessive because of immune complex mediated damage to the vessel wall. The proteins increase blood viscosity and may impair blood flow through capillaries. Retinal haemorrhages, central nervous system dysfunction, skin necrosis have all been described in this condition due to the marked elevation in the viscosity. In addition, these globulins may impair platelets adhesion and aggregation and interfere with fibrin polymerisation. The cryoglobulin comprises the cryoprecipitated Ig M; rheumatoid factor directed against endogenous Ig G.

B. To WHAT OTHER CONDITIONS MAY A LEUCOCYTOPLASTIC VASCULITIS PREDOMINANTLY INVOLVING THE SKIN, BE ASSOCIATED WITH?
ANS: This includes subacute bacterial endocarditis, Epstein-Barr virus infection, Chronic active hepatitis, ulcerative colitis, congenital deficiencies of various components, retroperitoneal fibrosis, primary biliary cirrhosis.

Association with hypersensitivity vasculitis with alpha 1 antitrypsin deficiency, intestinal bypass surgery and relapsing polychondritis has been described.

Leucocytoplastic vasculitis may also be associated with hairy cell leukaemia and classical polyarthritis nodosa.

C. HOW WOULD YOU TREAT THE PATIENT?
ANS: Eradication of the underlying infection, if possible, is of value in the therapy. Intermittent IV pulses of methyl prednisolone and intensive plasma exchange by the administration of glucocorticoids and cytotoxic agents, have been of value in severe cases.

Q 082

A 15-year-old son of an air craft engineer is brought in. They had just flown in from California. The child appears breathless and two sets of results were obtained four hours apart. The child was well prior to admission.

Results:
- PO_2 with 28%
- O_2 – 8.4 kPa
- PCO_2 – 5.7 kPa
- pH – 7.36
- Bicarbonate – 27 mmol/l

A. How would you manage this patient?

Ans: This patient has asthma and the rising PO_2 suggests he is getting tired and deteriorating towards respiratory failure. This patient needs to be transferred immediately to the intensive care unit. The British Thoracic Society guidelines suggest the severity of asthma is under diagnosed even by consultant physicians.

Q 083

The following results were obtained from a 41-year-old Indian cardiologist from Bhopal. He has a 2-month history of lethargy and recurrent headaches. This prevented him from studying for the USMILE and he is under a great deal of pressure to pass the examination as this is a prerequisite for employment. He is contemplating an arranged marriage in order to get a green card. His behaviour appears to be irrational at times and this has worsened over the last few weeks. He was found wandering aimlessly in the corridors of the Mass General Hospital on a Sunday, apparently lost.

Results:
• Sodium – 122 mmol/l
• Potassium – 4.1 mmol/l
• Urea – 7.7 mmol/l
• Creatinine – 97 μmol/l
• Bicarbonate – 22.3 mmol/l
• Glucose – 6.3 mmol/l
• Urine osmolality – 650 mosmol/kg
• CSF pressure – 23 cmHO
• CSF lymphocytes – 88 g/L
• CSF protein – 0.8 g/L
• CSF glucose – 2.9 mmol/l

A. What is the diagnosis?

Ans: This patient has TB meningitis and SIADH.

Q 084

A 48-year-old plastic surgeon is brought to the Accident and Emergency

Department shortly after Christmas. He had been found unconscious in his holiday caravan. The caravan was recently renovated and smells of solvent. He appears drowsy and complains of headache and is nauseous. He appears flushed and his temperature is 36.8°C. He also complains of a sense of feeling "lost at sea".

His respiratory rate is 23/min. An eye examination reveals visual field defects, blurred vision and venous engorgement with papilloedema. He complains of deafness in his right ear. Investigations show oxygen saturation by pulse oxymetry is normal.

A. WHAT IS THE DIAGNOSIS AND HOW SHOULD HE BE TREATED?

ANS: This patient has carbon monoxide poisoning from a defective heater.

Oxygen saturation by pulse oxymetry may be falsely normal. Deaths are common from carbon monoxide poisoning and occur usually prior to arrival to the hospital. Carbon monoxide is produced by the incomplete combustion of natural and tobacco products. Methylene chloride, a solvent in paint remover, is metabolised to carbon monoxide. This causes tissue hypoxia. Dissociation of the haemoglobin-carbon monoxide complex occurs, and carbon monoxide is excreted through the lungs.

In room air, the carbon monoxide half-life is 4–6 hours and decreases to 40–80 minutes when breathing 100% oxygen and 15–30 minutes with hyperbaric oxygen therapy. The apparent half-life after methylene chloride exposure is considerably longer.

B. WHAT ARE THE CARDIOVASCULAR MANIFESTATIONS OF THIS CONDITION?

ANS: It may include chest pain which is ischaemic, arrhythmia, heart failure and hypertension. Myoglobinuria secondary to muscle necrosis may result in renal failure and this may cause hypertension which may exacerbate the heart failure.

C. HOW WOULD YOU TREAT THIS PATIENT?

ANS: The patient should be removed from the site of exposure. Pure oxygen should be administered by a non-rebreathable mask at 10 L/min until carbon monoxide levels are less than 10% and all symptoms have resolved.

Endotracheal intubation and mechanical ventilation with 100%

oxygen are indicated in patients who have coma, significant brain dysfunction and cardiovascular instability. Hyperbaric oxygen at 2–3 atm prevents tissue hypoxia. A test for the carboxy haemoglobin level may be needed to document carbon monoxide exposure. Arrhythmia and hypotension are treated by usual measures. Pulmonary oedema (ARDS) can occur with carbon monoxide poisoning.

Carbon monoxide poisoning may lead to anoxic ischaemic encephalopathy. Patients with coma, syncope or seizures and those with signs or symptoms of neurological or cardiological dysfunction that do not resolve with oxygen or supportive therapy, are candidates for hyperbaric oxygen therapy. Hyperbaric oxygenation shortens the duration of coma and may prevent delayed sequalae. Should this patient need to be transferred by helicopter to a hyperbaric chamber the helicopter must fly at a low level.

D. WHAT OTHER CONDITIONS MAY LEAD TO THE SAME CEREBROVASCULAR DYSFUNCTION?

ANS: The other causes of anoxic ischaemic encephalopathy are myocardial infarction, cardiac arrest, a haemorrhage with shock and circulatory collapse (in these situations vascular supply to the brain is compromised before respiration), suffocation from drowning, strangulation, aspiration of vomitus or blood, compression of the trachea by haemorrhage or a surgical pad or a foreign body in the trachea, diseases that paralyse the muscles of respiration or compromise the CNS or respiratory drive, (traumatic vascular disease of the brain, epilepsy) causing respiratory failure followed by cardiac failure.

Q 085

A 26-year-old photojournalist for Time magazine was hit by an explosion while covering the border conflict of Pakistan and India. He is brought to the base hospital and the medical personnel do not find any localising neurological signs. A brain CT scan performed at the University hospital is reported to be normal.

- Sodium – 150 mmol/L
- Potassium – 3.2 mmol/L
- Urea – 8.3 mmol/L

- Creatinine – 82 μmol/L
- Bicarbonate – 25 mmol/L
- Glucose – 7.2 mmol/L
- Urine volume (12 hours) – 12 litres
- Osmolarity – 241 mosm/kg

A. WHAT IS THE DIAGNOSIS?
ANS: This patient has trauma induced cranial diabetes insipidus.
This may be treated with DDAVP (Desmopressin). It is interesting that DDAVP elevates the Von Willebrand factor and factor VIII and is an alternative treatment in both Willebrand factor deficiency and mild haemophilia. This was important in the early days prior to the improved purification of plasma products.

B. IS THERE A HEREDITARY FORM WHICH MAY PRODUCE A SIMILAR CONDITION?
ANS: X-linked nephrogenic diabetes insipidus. The kidney fails to respond to vasopressin and physiological studies indicate a defect in the V2 receptors. The gene for nephrogenic diabetes insipidus has been assigned to the q28-qtr portion of the X chromosome long arm by linkage and functional studies.

Other hereditary tubular defects such as juvenile nephronophthisis, medullary cystic and polycystic diseases, cystinosis and congenital or acquired urinary tract obstruction, may also cause vasopressin resistant diabetes insipidus. But in these syndromes, the characteristic features of the underlying disorders are also present. Affected infants become dehydrated easily, hypernatraemic and hyperthermic. This may damage the brain, causing retardation. In the absence of dehydration, overall renal function is normal. On intravenous urogram, the renal pelvis, ureters and bladder are dilated as in all forms of diabetes insipidus because of massive diuresis.

Q 086

A 69-year-old professor of ecology, who has been conducting a field study in anthropology in Peru, has been admitted on her return from South America. She complains of dry mouth and lack of salivation, diagnosed as Sjogren's syndrome. She also has vague complaints, of weakness. She is unmarried and lives alone. She lives on a diet consisting mainly of canned food.

On examination, she is emaciated. She is afebrile and has bruising on her arms. She has not had any falls. There is no lymphadenopathy and the abdominal examination is normal. She has mild pedal oedema.

Investigations:
- Hb – 9 g/dl
- MCV – 86 fl.
- MCHC – 33 g/dl
- WBC – 5 x 10^9/L
- Platelets – 160 x 10^9/L
- Reticulocytes – 6%
- Clotting studies – normal
- Bilirubin – 27 µmols/L
- LFT – normal
- Albumin – 23 g/dl
- Urine analysis – normal

A. WHAT IS THE DIAGNOSIS AND HOW WOULD YOU CONFIRM IT?
ANS: This lady has scurvy due to malnutrition. Vitamin C reduces the prosthetic metal ions in many enzymes to the required form and performs other antioxidant functions by removing free radicals.

The best understood function is the synthesis of collagen. Absence of the vitamin leads to the impairment of peptidyl hydroxylation of procollagen and a reduction in collagen formation and secretion by connective tissue. Nonhydroxylated collagen cannot form the triple helix required for normal tissue structure. Many features result from defect in collagen synthesis including the capillary fragility that underlies a haemorrhage, the poor healing of wounds, and bony abnormalities in children. Scorbutic patients excrete completely oxidised products of tyrosine, but the significance is unclear.

Symptoms do not improve until the pool is repleted. The larger the therapeutic dose, the faster the repletion. The assay of the leucocyte level of Vitamin C is diagnostic of scurvy.

B. WHAT ARE THE OTHER CLINICAL MANIFESTATIONS OF SCURVY?
ANS: Manifestation of clinical deficiency correlates better with total pool size than the plasma or blood levels.

The first symptoms of petechial haemorrhage and ecchymosis, correlate with a vitamin C pool size is less than 0.5 g. With further depletion, (pool size 0.1 – 0.5 g), manifestations include gum involvement, hyperkeratosis, congested hair follicles, arthralgia, Sjogren's syndrome (as in this patient), and joint effusion.

When depletion is extreme, (pool size less than 0.1 g), dyspnoea, edema, oliguria and neuropathy develop. Progress of the disease may then be rapid.

A 53-year-old karate instructor, has been treated for hypertension for the last seven years.

Her blood report:
• Sodium – 139 mmol/L
• Potassium – 2.9 mmol/L
• Urea – 13.1 mmol/L
• Creatinine – 143 μmol/L
• Plasma renin – increased

A. WHAT DIAGNOSIS WOULD YOU CONSIDER?
ANS:
i) Renal artery stenosis
Clinically, a bruit may be heard in the renal angle. The captopril induced renogram is highly specific and sensitive for the diagnosis of renal artery stenosis. This test utilises the dependency of the renal vasculature on angiotensin II. Individuals with renal artery stenosis are given a converting enzyme inhibitor (captopril) which reduces the angiotensin II level at the stenotic site. There will be renal blood flow pattern demonstrating a reduced uptake and delayed excretion as assessed by the isotope renogram. ACE inhibitors are contra-indicated as therapeutic agents in patients with bilateral renal artery stenosis or a unilateral renal artery stenosis with a solitary functioning kidney. The gold standard of surgically correctable renal disease is a combination of renal angiography and renal vein determination. The renal angiogram establishes the presence of renal artery stenosis and determines whether it is due to arteriosclerosis or fibromuscular dysplasia. The presence

of renal artery stenosis does not prove the lesion is responsible for the hypertension nor does it predict the chances of a surgical cure as renal artery stenosis is a frequent finding in normotensive individuals during post-mortem. Essential hypertension is common and may occur in combination with renal artery stenosis - this may not be responsible for the hypertension.

Bilateral renal vein catheterisation to measure plasma renin activity is therefore used to assess the functional significance of any lesions noted by arteriography. The ischaemic kidney has a higher venous renin level by a factor of 1.5 or more. The renal venous blood draining a normal kidney exhibit levels similar to those in the IVC below the entrance of the renal veins.

Significant benefit from operative correction may be anticipated in at least 80% of patients with the findings described above if impeccable preparation is performed prior to renal vein blood sampling. This preparation includes discontinuing renin suppressing agents, such as beta blockers, for at least a week and putting the patient on a low sodium diet for four days. When obstructing lesions in the branches of the renal arteries are revealed by arteriography, an attempt to obtain blood samples from the main branches of the renal veins should be made in an effort to identify a localised intraarterial lesion responsible for the hypertension.

ii) Diuretic induced dehydration

iii) A rennin secreting tumour
Secondary aldosteronism with hypertension may be caused, rarely, by a renin producing tumour in primary reninism. These patients have the biochemical characteristics of renal vascular hypertension. The defect is in renin secretion by a juxtaglomerular cell tumour.

The diagnosis can be made by the absence of changes in venal vasculature, demonstration of space-occupying lesions in the kidney by radiographic techniques, and documentation of unilateral increase in renal vein renin activity. Rarely do these tumors arise from tissues such as the ovary. A rare form of renal hypertension results from the excess secretion of renin by the juxtaglomerular cell tumor or nephroblastomas. In contrast to primary aldosteronism, peripheral renin activity is elevated instead of subnormal. This disease can be distinguished from other forms of secondary aldosteronism by the presence of normal renal function and with unilateral increase in renal renin concentration without a renal artery lesion.

Q 088

A 24-year-old soldier has a 4-year history of diarrhoea, up to five times a day. There is no rectal bleeding. He complains of intermittent abdominal discomfort and a weight loss of 7 kg over the last six months. He has suffered recurrent ulceration of his tongue for several years. He has felt under the weather during the preceding four months and complains of a vague sense of weakness and lethargy; he was finding his field trips and weapons difficult to bear. He is on no medication and has no significant medical history. He smokes 30 cigarettes and drinks 5–9 units of alcohol daily.

On examination, he is a short man with angular stomatitis and there are some aphthous ulcers in the oral cavity. He has mild proximal weakness and feels an uncomfortable pressure on both the sacral iliac joints.

Investigation:
- Hb – 9.1 g/dl
- MCV – 100 fl
- WBC – 9 x 10^9/L
- Platelets – 175 x 10^9/L
- Peripheral smear – macrocytes, target cells and Howell-Jolly bodies
- Potassium – 2.9 mmols/L
- ALP – 170 IU/L
- Total proteins – 56 g/dl
- Albumin – 24 g/dl
- Corrected calcium – 1.8 mmols/L
- Phosphate – 0.8 mmols/L
- Urea, electrolytes, LFT – normal
- Fecal fat – 35 mmols/day

A. WHAT IS THE DIAGNOSIS AND HOW WOULD YOU EXPLAIN THE ABNORMAL HAEMATOLOGICAL INDICES?
ANS: This patient has coeliac disease with hyposplenism (as evidenced

by target cells and Howell-Jolly bodies). He has also got osteomalacia due to malabsorption. The macrocytosis may either be due to folate deficiency or may be alcohol induced.

Coeliac disease in children and coeliac sprue in adults are one and the same disorder with the same pathogenesis. The discordance for coeliac sprue among HLA identical siblings and identical twins raises the possibility of an additional susceptibility gene(s) which has yet to be identified.

This patient should be put on a gluten free diet as this will reduce the degree of malabsorption and prevent gut damage. The diagnosis may be proved by jejunal biopsy which will demonstrate blunting of intestinal villi and a lymphoma which may manifest itself occasionally as weight-loss and abdominal pain. This may be diagnosed by CT scan, small bowel enema and laparoscopy.

Q 089

A 27-year-old Chinese film director has a 2-week history of pedal oedema and frothy urine. He has been having night sweats, and intermittent pruritis which he ascribes to the weather and weightloss. He has no significant medical history and is not on any medication.

On examination, he has left supraclavicular and axillary lymphadenopathy. The pulse is regular at 86/min, lying BP 150/80 mmHg and standing BP 156/91 mmHg, and the neck veins are not elevated. He has marked sacral oedema and there is no visceromegaly palpable.

Investigation:
- Hb – 11 g/d1
- WBC – 10.5 x 10^9/L
- Platelets – 300 x 10^9/L
- Sodium – 143 mmols/L
- Potassium – 3.8 mmols/L
- Urea – 3.7 mmols/L
- Creatinine – 97 mmols/L
- Total proteins – 40 g/d1
- Albumin – 19 g/dl
- Urine protein – ++++++
- Urine blood – negative

- Inactive sediment
- 24-hours urine protein excretion – 9.2 g
- Creatinine clearance – 42 mls/min
- CXR – normal
- Abdominal ultrasound – marginally enlarged kidneys

A. WHAT IS THE MOST LIKELY DIAGNOSIS?
ANS: This patient has Stage II b Hodgkin's lymphoma with nephrotic syndrome.

The histology of this renal pathology is usually minimal change lesion. The mechanism of the association of Hodgkin's disease with minimal change disease may involve an underlying T-cell abnormality. Proteinuria waxes and wanes with fluctuation in the clinical activity of the Hodgkin's disease.

Remission may be produced by local irradiation of involved lymph nodes or by systemic chemotherapy.

Q 090

A 37-year-old jet fighter pilot, who smokes heavily, complains of increasing unsteadiness over the preceding six months. He is unable to fly and has been moved to a desk job. He is now deaf in his left ear, which he attributes to the high frequency sounds of the jet. The airforce physician had diagnosed a left sided Bell's palsy.

On examination, he has a wide based ataxic gait with normal light touch, vibration and proprioception in the lower limbs. He has a left sensorineural deafness and an LMN left 7th nerve palsy. The left corneal reflex is absent and he has never used contact lenses.

Investigation:
- Full blood count, urea, electrolytes, LFT's, and the skull X-rays – normal,
- Chest X-ray – dextrocardia with no situs inversus
- ESR – 20 mm/hour

A. WHAT IS THE DIAGNOSIS AND WHAT INVESTIGATION WOULD CONFIRM THIS?
ANS: This patient has a left cerebellopontine angle tumour which may be caused by an Acoustic Schwanomma (neuroma).

There is an association between neurofibromatosis type II, carried on chromosome 22, an autosomal dominant disorder in which neurofibroma involves the acoustic nerves specifically and bilateral involvement is common.

Acoustic neurinomas may produce deafness and symptoms of a cerebellopontine angle lesion. They may also be associated with meningiomas and astrocytomas. An asymmetric but conjugate horizontal gaze evolved nystagmus occurs with unilateral cerebellar disease and cerebellopontine angle tumours such as acoustic neuroma or a meningioma.

Q 091

A 54-year-old Scottish nanny to a single mother of four children was referred for investigation of episodes of fainting. She tended to faint easily as a girl and was not allowed to undergo physical exercise in school. Her condition has worsened in the past six months. Now she suffers from dizzy spells lasting for about three minutes. These spells occur when she stands up too quickly, and she feels faint when she stands for more than a few minutes over the stove. She gives no history of palpitations, precordial discomfort or shortness of breath. Over the past six years, she has experienced an increase in the frequency of urination, with urge incontinence. She complains of constipation and this has gotten worse during the last few weeks. She has also become clumsy and burnt herself while in the kitchen.

On examination, her skin is dry (although she uses emollient creams regularly.) Her pulse is 64/min, regular, the lying BP 130/80 mmHg and the sitting BP 90/68 mmHg and the standing (when she looked rather pale) BP 84/46 mmHg. The neck veins are not elevated and heart sounds are normal. There is no bruit on auscultation. There is no oedema. She has dysarthria and appears unsteady when walking.

Investigation:
- Full blood count – normal
- Urea and electrolytes – normal
- LFT – normal
- ECG – within normal limits

A. What is the diagnosis?

Ans: This patient has multisystem atrophy with autonomic neuropathy (the Shy-Drager syndrome).

Bradbury and Eggleston in 1925 described the combination of postural hypotension, incontinence, impotence and abnormalities of sweating. Symptoms of central neurological origin develop later, comprising predominantly extrapyramidal or cerebellar dysfunction.

In 1960, Shy and Drager described neuropathological changes in the brain stem and basal ganglia. Subsequently, other researchers have spotted a prominent loss of neurons in central regions of the autonomic nervous system. This condition affects cells in the intermediolateral column of the thoracic spinal cord. Abnormalities have also been found in the peripheral autonomic ganglia, due to cellular loss. Cell-loss is accompanied by gliosis. Lewy bodies typical of Parkinson's disease are present in some cases. In patients in whom Parkinsonism progresses more rapidly than idiopathic Parkinson's disease, akinesia, rigidity and postural disturbances, but not tremors, are prominent. If there is no improvement with L-dopa, the diagnosis of striatonigral degeneration should be considered.

Usually it is not possible to distinguish with certainty between striatonigral degeneration from idiopathic Parkinson's disease or other akinetic rigid syndromes. Unfortunately, confirmation of a clinical diagnosis of striatonigral degeneration can only be made by post-mortem examination.

Many neurologists consider the Shy-Drager syndrome to be a unique form of multisystem degeneration, resembling but distinct from either Parkinson's disease or OPCA (Olivopontocerebellar-atrophy). Anhydrosis is common and can be demonstrated by placing the individual in a warm room after the application of a starched-iodine mixture to the skin. Cerebellar gait ataxia may be evident.

MRI may demonstrate a T2 weighted signal hypointensity in the putamen, globus pallidus and *substantia nigra*. Positron emission tomography shows a decreased uptake of dopamine derivative in the putamen and caudate, probably reflecting a loss of nigrostriatal dopaminergic neurons.

B. How would you treat this patient?

Ans: Treatment is symptomatic. The postural hypotension is usually the most disabling symptom.

Antigravity stockings to minimise pooling of venous blood in the legs are recommended. A leotard that covers the lower abdomen may provide additional benefit. Increase salt intake combined with fluorohydrocortisone may be beneficial. In severe cases, adrenergic drugs such as ephedrine, L-dopa or amphetamine may improve the disability.

The Parkinson's symptoms often respond initially to Bromocryptine or Sinemet (carbidopa-levodopa), but later in the course most patients become resistant to these agents. Centrally acting alpha agonist, e.g. Yohimbine or Clonidine may be beneficial.

The patient should be advised to stay in the shade during summer or when in the tropics.

Q 092

A 72-year-old Supreme Court judge is admitted to hospital complaining of bright red rectal bleeding. He complains of several mild episodes of rectal bleeding where he was told he had piles. He was treated by an alternative medicine healer with no success.

On examination, he appears pale with cold fingers. Pulse rate is 110/min, regular and lying BP 120/80 mmHg, sitting BP 105/78 mmHg. An abdominal examination does not reveal any visceromegaly, while a rectal examination reveals some clotted blood. Proctoscopy and sigmoidoscopy are normal.

Investigation:
- Hb – 8.7 g/dl
- MCV – 73 fl
- WBC – 8 x 10^9/L
- Platelets – 550 x 10^9/L
- Sodium – 138 mmols/L
- Potassium – 4.3 mmols/L
- Urea – 5.7 mmols/L
- Creatinine – 123 µmols/L
- LFT – normal
- Barium studies – normal

A. WHAT IS THE MOST LIKELY DIAGNOSIS?
ANS: This patient has angiodysplasia of the colon.

This vascular ectasia (not neoplasm), which occurs in the colon of older individuals, may cause bleeding. Aortic stenosis occurs in some patients and may cause chronic ischaemia leading to angiodysplasia. Gross angiodysplasia looks similar to spider angiomas on the skin and appear as star-shaped branching vessels in the submucosa measuring up to 2 mm in diameter. The lesions are usually multiple and are found mainly in the caecum and ascending colon, but in some patients they may be distributed from the stomach to the rectum.

The diagnosis is easily established by colonoscopy, which allows treatment by electrocautery or injection with a sclerosant. Some patients with uncontrolled bleeding or with multiple sites of angiodysplasia may require a right hemicolectomy. Angiodysplasias may also respond to chronic oestrogen and progesterone therapy.

B. WHAT OTHER CONDITIONS MAY HAVE CAUSED BLEEDING IN THE PATIENT?
ANS: Cancer of the colon, polyps and ulcerative colitis are common causes. It is less frequent in granulomatous colitis, but occult blood may be present in the stool. Bleeding may accompany infection with Shigella, amoeba, campylobacter, clostridium difficile and, rarely, salmonella.

In the elderly, ischaemic colitis may be a cause of frank bloody diarrhoea. Ischaemic colitis can be seen in younger women who use oral contraceptive pills.

Q 093

A 21-year-old interior designer is found unconscious near the swimming pool, after an argument with her ex-husband. She has been on medication for postherpetic neuralgia. She appears drowsy on admission, but groans and grimaces to pressure on the supraorbital region. Her eyes do not open and she flexes her limbs symmetrically to painful stimulus applied to her nails. Muscle tone is normal and tendon reflexes are depressed. Her plantar responses are equivocal. Her pupils are dilated equally on both sides and react briskly to light. She has a divergent strabismus and absent oculocephalic and oculovestibular reflexes. The optic fundus is normal. Her temperature is 36.3°C and she has a sinus tachycardia of 124/min with a BP of 94/60 mmHg.

A. What is the probable diagnosis of her condition?

Ans: This patient has a tricyclic antidepressant overdose which has produced broad complex tachycardia – either a ventricular or supraventricular tachycardia with a bundle branch block.

Antidepressants are the fourth most common cause of drug overdose seen in emergency departments in the U.S., and is the third most common cause of drug-related death after alcohol-drug combination and heroin. In a California study (Callaham and Kassel) the annual frequency of tricyclic overdose was 1.3/100,000 population. More than 2/3 of the victims were women. Amitryptylline, Desipramine and Nortryptyline are the most commonly used drugs. The tricyclic antidepressants are extremely useful for management of patients with chronic pain. Although developed for the treatment of depression, the tricyclics have a dose related biological activity for the production of analgesia in a variety of clinical conditions. The mechanism of this activity is unknown. The analgesic effect of tricyclic has a more rapid action and this occurs at a lower dose than is typically required for the treatment of depression. Furthermore, patients with chronic pain, who are not depressed, obtain pain relief with tricyclic antidepressants.

There is evidence that tricyclic drugs potentiate opioid analgesia, so they are useful adjuncts for the therapy of persistent pain such as those that occurs with malignancy. The tricyclics that have been shown to relieve pain have significant side-effects. Unfortunately, some of the newer antidepressants such as flouoxetine (Prozac), that have fewer and less serious side-effects, have not been shown to provide pain relief although they are safer in the long run. Many physicians are unaware that the tricyclics are used for the relief of chronic painful conditions and one should not assume that all patients who are on tricyclic antidepressants are non-compos mentis.

The tricyclic antidepressants, especially imipramine, have a quinidine like action and may produce cardiac arrhythmias. This has been associated with sudden death in a few patients. It is paradoxical that one should give a potentially life-threatening drug to a patient who is depressed and may have suicidal ideas. It is interesting that in some instances the quinidine like action has been used advantageously, with a once daily dosing in experimental trials, to produce antiarrhythmic effects. Imipramine has been used by pharmaceutical companies as a comparison drug for other type Ia antiarrhythmics.

The most bothersome symptoms from the anticholinergic effects, do cause discomfort and compliance problems. Despite the problems, the risk-benefit ratio is overwhelmingly in favour of this class of antidepressants and thousands of patients have been treated with these compounds safely and effectively.

Death from dysrhythmias occurs within 2–6 hours following intoxication. Prolongation of the QRS complex (greater than 100 msecs) in severe overdoses correlate with an increased risk of cardiac arrhythmias and with seizures. Serum levels should be taken and are diagnostic. The level correlates with the severity. Metabolites, as well as the parent compound level, should be added together when estimating the serum concentration. A level over 3,300 nmols/L (1,000 ng/ml) indicates serious poisoning and is associated with QRS complexes wider than 100 msecs.

B. How should this patient be treated?

Ans: Ipecac induced emesis is contraindicated with tricyclic ingestion. Gastric lavage is contra-indicated in tricyclic ingestion. Gastric lavage is indicated for comatose patients with recent ingestion. Activated charcoal in single or repeated doses should be administered. Treatment includes support of respiration and volume expansion, and the ventricular tachyarrhythmia should be treated appropriately by using sodium bicarbonate, lidocaine and phenytoin. Beta adrenergic blockers and Class Ia antiarrhythmics eg. Quinidine, procainamide and disopyramide should be avoided.

Cardiac pacing may be necessary for the severely depressed myocardium. Correction of acidosis is an important component of the treatment of cardiac arrhythmias and seizures. Physostigmine will reverse low dose anticholinergic effects and may be administered in mild poisoning if deterioration has been excluded by a suitable period of observation. Physostigmine can cause asystole in severe poisoning and should not be used in this situation. It is an absolute contraindication in dysrhythmias as in the case described or in cardiac conduction disturbances. Hence cardiac monitoring and defibrillation should be immediately available.

The first six hours after a tricyclic antidepressant overdose is known as the Golden hour as this is crucial for therapy. CNS depression and seizures, respiratory arrest and cardiovascular arrhythmias are the principle causes of death. ECG changes showing prolongation of QRS are early signs of toxicity and ventricular fibrillation is a common complication. ECG changes are a more sensitive measurement for treating patients than are blood levels of the drug.

C. WHAT OTHER PAINFUL CONDITIONS MAY RESPOND TO THE CHEMICAL AGENT USED TO TREAT THIS PATIENT'S INTRACTABLE PAINFUL POSTHERPETIC NEURALGIA? ANS: The tricyclic antidepressants have been shown in control trials to demonstrate analgesia in diabetic neuropathy, tension headache, migraine headache, cancer and rheumatoid arthiritis. Control studies indicate benefit, but not analgesia for chronic low back pain.

Q 094

A 27-year-old swimming instructor, a former national swimmer, has recovered recently from a non-specific viral infection. She is admitted to the hospital with a 5-day history of increasing oliguria with headaches and nose bleeds. She feels tired, vomited during the examination and has had a number of petechial rashes for the last three days. There is no significant medical history, but she took anabolic steroids in her teens while preparing for competitive swimming. She specialised in the 100 m freestyle. She is engaged to a Mathematics teacher and has been on the contraceptive pill for the last eight months.

On examination, she is afebrile, there is no palpable lymphadenopathy. Pulse 90/min regular. JVP is raised 3 cm, BP 184/120 mmHg with normal heart sounds and pedal oedema. There is a purpuric rash on the limbs.

Investigation:
- Hb – 7.8 g/dl
- WBC – 7.2 x 10⁹/L
- Platelets – 34 x 10⁹/L
- Reticulocytes – 2.3%
- Blood film – target cells, schizocytes with no Rouleux formation
- Clotting studies – normal
- Fibrinogen – 1.5 g/L (N-2-4)
- Coomb's test – negative
- Haptoglobin – absent
- Sodium – 143 mmols/L

- Potassium – 6.3 mmols/L
- Standard bicarbonate – 15 mmols/L
- Urea – 43 mmols/L
- Creatinine – 910 micromols/L
- Urine protein – +++
- Urine blood – +++
- Occasional granular cast and RBCs
- ECG and CXR – within normal limits

A. WHAT IS THE DIAGNOSIS?

ANS: This patient has the haemolytic uraemic syndrome.

The aetiological factors may be either of a viral nature or, rarely, the disorder appears to be familial in nature. The haemolytic uraemic syndrome (HUS) resembles TTP. As in TTP, there is no evidence of disseminated intravascular coagulation. In contrast to TTP, in HUS the disorder remains localised in the kidney, where hyaline thrombi are seen in the afferent arterioglomerular capillaries. Such thrombi are not present in other vessels and neurological symptoms, other than those associated with uraemia, are uncommon.

There is no effective therapy. However, dialysis for acute renal failure has reduced the initial mortality to only 5%. Between 10–15% of patients are left with chronic renal impairment. Typically, the LDH level is elevated, indicating intravascular haemolysis. The benefits of antiplatelet drugs (aspirin, dipyridamole, and FFP) are unclear, but they are commonly used. H antigens, proteins found on bacterial flagella, are linked to the haemolytic uraemic syndrome (ie sero-group 0157:H7).

The haemolytic uraemic syndrome is also associated with other bacteria other that 0157:H7, such as other E.coli sero-types and shigella. There is also some evidence that some enteropathogenic viruses and Rotavirus may participate in the pathogenesis of the haemolytic uraemic syndrome and idiopathic acute nephritis. The haematological abnormality is microangiopathic haemolytic anaemia (MAHA). A disorder resembling the haemolytic uraemic syndrome has been described in adults treated with the neoplastic drug Mitomycin C, usually in combination with other drugs.

Q 095

A 70-year-old Professor of Physics, who works on the nuclear reactor programme of the Indian subcontinent, is admitted to hospital with a 2-day history of dry cough, increasing shortness of breath, fever, rigor and a right sided pleuritic thoracic pain. He complains of a vague discomfort over the left abdominal region. He has lost a great deal of weight and claims he has been skipping meals in his involvement in the building of a reactor. He has lost 4 kg over the last six months.

On examination, he is febrile at 38.5°C, sweating profusely and cervical lymph nodes are palpable. His pulse rate is 100/min; BP 130/80 mmHg and he also has some cold sores. He is breathing rapidly with a respiratory rate of 29/min and there is bronchial breathing with a few crackles in the right lung base. A firm 3-fingers-breath liver is palpable with a 4-finger-breath spleen below the left costal margin.

Investigation:
- Hb – 9 g/dl
- MCV – 91 fl
- WBC – 38×10^9/L (There is a marked increase in granulocytes with a left shift in differentiation, including an increase in myelocytes, promyelocytes and metamyelocytes; eosinophilia and basophilia are prominent.)
- Platelets – 320×10^9/L
- ESR – 60 mm/h
- CRP – 100 mg/L (Normal 0–10)
- Urea – normal
- Electrolytes – normal
- LFT – normal
- Clotting profile – normal
- Neutrophil alkaline phosphatase score – low
- CXR (PA and lateral views) – consolidation in the right lower lobe and pleural effusion.

A. What are the two likely diagnoses?

Ans: Radiation induced chronic myeloid leukaemia and pneumococcal pneumonia.

Chronic mycloid leukaemia is a clonal stem disorder characterised by an increase in myeloid activity and the presence of the Philadelphia chromosome. The Philadelphia chromosome involves the translocation of the Abelson (abl) proto-oncogene on chromosome 9 to the break point cluster region (BCR) of chromosome 22 with the formation of a fusion gene called BCR-abl. CML is an acquired disorder and was observed in survivors of the atomic bomb explosions in Hiroshima and Nagasaki. The peak incidence of CML is seen 5–12 years after radiation exposure and appears to be dose related. The Philadelphia chromosome is present in virtually all patients with CML and in 1/4 of adults and 5% of children with acute lymphoblastic leukaemia.

Pneumococcal pneumonia usually improves promptly when appropriate antimicrobial therapy is given. Within 12–24 hours after initiation of therapy with penicillin, the temperature, pulse and respiration should begin to fall and may normalise. The temperature of half the patients requires four days or longer to become normal, and failure of the temperature to do so in 1–2 days should not prompt a change in antibacterial therapy in the absence of other indications. A return of physical findings in the lungs to normal after pneumoccal pneumonia, usually takes place in 2–4 weeks. X-ray evidence of residual pulmonary consolidation, however, may persist as long as eight weeks, and other radiological manifestation of the infection may persist up to 18 weeks. The process of resolution may require a longer time in those over 50 years and in those with chronic obstructive airway disease.

A lung abscess is a rare sequel to pneumococcal infection, although pneumococcal pneumonia is not an uncommon complication to a lung abscess of other origins. Lung abscess is manifested by continual fever, profuse expectoration of purulent sputum and the X-ray shows one or more cavities. This complication is exceedingly rare in patients who have received penicillin therapy and is most likely to follow infection with pneumococcus type 3. Pleural effusion is detectable in approximately half the patients with pneumococcal pneumonia and is associated with a delay in initiation of therapy and bacteraemia. Usually the effusion is sterile and is absorbed spontaneously within a week or two. At times the effusion is large and requires aspiration of drainage.

Before the era of effective chemotherapy, empyema occurred in up to 8% of patients with pneumococcal pneumonia. It is now observed in less than 1% of treated cases. It manifests clinically by persistent fever or pleuritic pain, together with signs of pleural effusion. In the early stages, the gross appearance of infected fluid may not differ from that of sterile pleural effusion. Later, there is profuse outpouring of polymorpholeucocytes and fibrin, resulting in exudate of thick greenish pus containing large clots of fibrin. The quantity of exudate may be large enough to displace mediastinal structure. In neglected cases, this process leads to extensive pleural scarring, with limitation of thoracic movement. Rupture and drainage through the chest wall may occur, but is rare. A metastatic brain abscess is an occasional complication of empyema.

Q 096

A 75-year-old member of parliament complains of a feeling of transient dizziness during which he feels weak and is unable to speak. For three years he has experienced bouts of generalised weakness and dizziness, occurring every three months and lasting for about eight minutes. These episodes were not related to a change in the pattern of micturation, coughing or sudden neck movements. He has never fallen or lost consciousness during the attacks, and is not on any medication. His secretary, who had witnessed the last episode, noticed the patient was pale at onset of the attack and flushed on recovery.

On examination, he appears to be well. His pulse rate is 74/min and his blood pressure is 120/80 mmHg. There is no postural drop. No abnormal heart sounds are heard and carotid bruit is not audible. The full blood count, urea, electrolytes and blood sugar are all normal. The resting ECG is reported as normal.

A. What is the description given to the episodes the patient is experiencing and what are the possible causes?

Ans: The patient is experiencing Stokes-Adams attacks.

This may be due to a disease of the sinus node, the sick sinus syndrome, ischaemic heart disease or even a cardiomyopathy. He should undergo a 24-hour Holter monitor and a cardiomemo which may sometimes be temporarily be implantable. He should also undergo a stress test, utilising the Bruce protocol to seek out ischaemic heart disease involving the right coronary artery system.

Should the Holter document episodes of AV block, ventricular asystole, sinus bradycardia, sinoatrial block, sinus arrest, sick sinus syndrome, carotid syncope or episodic ventricular tachycardia with or without associated brady arrhythmias, one should pace the patient with a DDD pacemaker. The DDD pacemaker allows atrioventricular synchrony. VVI pacemakers should not be routinely used in relatively healthy patients as the asynchronous pacing mode predisposes to atrial fibrillation, which in turn increases the propensity for strokes.

In the classical Stokes-Adams attack, the patient is warned of the impending faint by a sense of "feeling bad". A sense of giddiness and movement or swaying of the floor or surrounding objects ensues. The senses become confused, the patient yawns or gapes and there are spots before the eyes. The vision may dim and the ear may ring. Nausea and, sometimes, vomiting accompany these symptoms. There is a striking pallor or ashen-gray colour of the face as in this patient. Very often, the face and body are bathed in cold perspiration. In some patients, a deliberate onset may allow time for protection against injury. In others, the occurrence of syncope is sudden and without warning.

In a patient with faintness or syncope attended by bradycardia, one has to distinguish between a failure of neurogenic reflexes to maintain blood pressure from that to a cardiogenic Stokes-Adams attack. The ECG is decisive, but even without it, the Stokes-Adams attack can be recognised clinically by their longer duration, by the pattern of bradycardia, by the presence of audible sounds synchronous with atrial contractions, by atrial contractions (A waves in the JVP), and by marked variation in intensity of the first heart-sound despite the regular rhythm. In some patients, ventricular tachycardia or fibrillation may follow a period of asystole, resulting in syncope or sudden death. For patients with syncope and suspected sinus node dysfunction for which the diagnosis is not established by ambulatory ECG recording, electrophysiological testing may be helpful in unmasking diagnostic abnormalities. It is remarkable that this Stokes Adams syndrome was diagnosed before the discovery of the ECG and is a testament of clinical observation.

A 64-year-old marble sculptor, an outpatient, has a five month history of progressive swelling of the right arm, increasing dyspnoea and a persistent dry cough. His voice has also become hoarse over the same period and he has lost a great deal of weight. He smokes up to 15 cigarettes a day.

On examination, he appears emaciated and cannot speak above a whisper. He is dyspnoeic at rest and his right arm is swollen with dilated veins on the right shoulder and the right side of the upper thorax. There is dullness on percussion and reduced air entry in the right upper zone of the chest with ptosis of the right eye. All tendon reflexes are depressed in the right arm, but it is difficult to determine this due to the swelling.

A. WHAT IS THE DIAGNOSIS?

ANS: This patient has a Pancoast tumour which a chest X-ray will confirm by demonstrating an apical shadowing, rib erosion and consolidation. There would be a zone of local atelectasis.

Pancoast syndrome is due to carcinoma of the superior pulmonary sulcus, often treated with radiotherapy and surgery. This patient should have the usual pre-operative staging procedure, including mediastinoscopy and CT scan to determine tumour extent and a neurological examination with electromyography to document neurologic findings. Histologic diagnosis is not usually made, and with the constellation of tumour location and pain distribution, the diagnostic accuracy is better than 90%. If mediastinoscopy is negative, two curative approaches may be used in treating the pancoast tumour.

In the first, preoperative irradiation (3,000 rad/30 Gy in 10 treatments) is given to the area, followed by an enblock resection of the tumour and involved chest wall 3–6 weeks later. At three years, survival figures of 42% for epidermoid and 21% for adenoma and large cell carcinoma have been reported.

The second approach involves radiotherapy alone in curative doses with a similar survival-rate to that of combine modality therapy. Steroids may be used to reduce the swelling of the arm. Non-invasive Doppler techniques are helpful especially in evaluating the vascular supply of the region.

Q 098

A 32-year-old Imam of a mosque is admitted after collapsing during a prayer session. He normally enjoys good health, but did fall into a hole while walking around archeological sites in the region of Mecca. He was well until ten hours prior to admission, when he developed malaise, anorexia, vomiting and diarrhoea. He has rigors and complains of intractable leg pain.

On examination, he is flushed with a temperature of 38.8°C, pulse 120/min regular; blood pressure peripheries are warm. The gash on his right arm is noted and the surrounding area is reddened, indurated and tender. An X-ray of the arm does not reveal any feature suggestive of either osteomyelitis or gas gangrene.

- Hb – 15.3 g/dl
- WBC – 13 x 10^9/L with a marked shift on the left in the WBC differential with many immature granulocytes.
- Platelets – 98 x 10^9/L
- ESR – 100 mm/h
- Sodium – 143 mmol/L
- Potassium – 4.3 mmol/L
- Urea – 8.7 mmol/L
- Creatinine – 82 µmol/L
- ALT – 198 IU/L
- AST – 110 IU/L
- Albumin – 42 g/L
- Urinalysis – normal
- Chest X-ray – normal.
- The ECG – shows sinus tachycardia, but otherwise normal.

A. WHAT IS THE DIAGNOSIS?

ANS: This patient has septicaemia from cellulitis, which has produced the streptococcal toxic shock-like syndrome.

This was described in 1987 by Conns and associates in association with patients with group A streptococcal infection which had manifested as a multi system disease characterized by shock. It is called the streptococcal toxic shock-like syndrome because it shares certain features with staphylococcal toxic shock syndrome. While a formal case definition has not been established, the general features of the syndrome include fever, hypotension, renal impairment and respiratory distress syndrome.

A majority of patients with streptococcal syndrome are bacteraemic. The most common associated infection is a soft tissue infection-necrotising fasciitis, myositis or cellulitis, although a variety of local infections have been described in association with the syndrome, including pneumonia, peritonitis, osteomyelitis and myositis.

Streptococcal toxic shock-like syndrome is associated with 30% mortality, with most deaths due to shock and respiratory failure. Because of the rapid downhill nature of the disease, early diagnosis is essential. Patients should be aggressively supported in the form of fluid resuscitation, vasopressor infusion and mechanical ventilation. In addition to anti-microbial therapy, and in cases associated with necrotising fasciitis, surgical debridement can also be used. The syndrome has been strongly associated with the production of a pyogenic exotoxin A.

In light of the possible role of this or other streptococcal toxins in streptococcal toxic shock-like syndrome, treatment of patients with clindamycin has been advocated by some authorities who argue that through its direct action on protein synthesis, clindamycin is more effective than penicillin, a cell-wall agent, in rapidly terminating toxin production. Support of this view comes from studies of an experimental model of streptococcal myositis, in which mice treated with clindamycin had improved survival over those that receive penicillin.

Comparable data for the treatment of human infection is not available. One may treat the patient with a combination of benzyl penicillin, flucloxacillin and gentarnycin as an alternative. Blood cultures and wound swabs should be taken for culture and sensitivity. The coagulation screen should be performed.

Q 099

A 27-year-old ornithologist, who travels widely in South America, has fever, rash, lymphadenopathy and oral ulceration. He is currently on no medication and has been studying the pattern of bird migration because of the danger of the spread of Avian flu. He underwent a full course of treatment for primary syphilis a year ago. He has been well, apart from nephritic syndrome which resolved spontaneously six months ago and denies any history of sexual contact. He claims he has been celibate since the diagnosis which psychologically traumatised him. He has repeated the test for syphilis as he is planning to get married and gaining the right of abode in America. The laws and regulations of the state require routine premarital testing for syphilis.

Investigation:
- VDRL – positive; 1/10
- TPHA – positive
- FTA – positive

A. WHAT ARE THE TWO POSSIBLE INTERPRETATIONS FOR THE DATA?
ANS: This patient has reinfection and has secondary syphilis.

The nephritic syndrome, in early congenital syphilis as in adult syphilis, represents an immune complex induced glomerulonephritis. It is possible false positive VDRL may be caused by other infections such as infectious mononucleosis, and inflammatory causes such as SLE.

One should aspirate the lymph node for dark ground microscopy to search for the spirochete. A meatal sore may be used to sample for dark ground microscopy. TPHA and the FTA are positive for life after syphilis. Examination of oral lesions by dark field technique is not recommended as it is difficult to differentiate treponema pallidum from other spirochetes that may be present in the oral cavity. Other treponemal species are found in the mouth, genital mucosa and gastrointestinal tract, but have no pathogenic role. This can be confused with treponema pallidum on dark field examination. An oral treponema in coal workers was described by Riviere. This organism is very closely related to treponemapallidum antigenically and is significantly associated with periodontitis and acute necrotising ulcerative gingivitis. Its aetiological role in this gum disease is known. A single negative dark field examination does not exclude the diagnosis. Most syphilis is diagnosed in private clinics where dark field microscopy is not available.

Other means of identification for treponema pallidum in exudates is needed. The direct fluorescent antibody treponema pallidum (DFA-TP) test is available. Laboratories use fluorescein-conjugated polyclonal anti-treponemal antibody for detection of treponema in fixed smears prepared from suspect lesions. Because of cross-reactive antibodies which will also stain commencial non-pathogenic spirochetes, the antiserum is extensively absorbed with culture treponems in an effort to produce a specific reagent. A refinement of this technique using a monoclonal antibody specific to the pathogenic treponems has been developed, but is not yet available widely. It is as sensitive and as specific as dark field microscopy for the examination of suspicious lesions.

A new monoclonal antibody-based ELISA test, which detects

treponema pallidum in swab specimens from primary and secondary lesions, is currently being evaluated. The presence of specific Ig M antibody may be used as a marker for active syphilis. Theoretically the Ig M should disappear following adequate therapy. The rate at which Ig M drops after therapy is variable from patient to patient and the use of these criteria for cure is not accepted by all.

Penicillin G is the drug of choice for stages of syphilis. Treponema pallidum is killed by very low concentrations of penicillin G, although a long period of antibiotics is required for treatment because of the unusually slow rate of multiplication of the organism. The efficacy of penicillin for syphilis remains undiminished after half a century of use. Other antibiotic choices include the tetracyclines, erythromycin and the cephalosporins. Aminoglycosids and spectinomycin inhibits treponema pallidum only very large doses and the sulfonamides and the quinolones are not active against them.

The optimal dose and duration of the therapy has not been established for any stage of syphilis. The recurrence rate of a regimen increases as infection progresses from incubating syphilis to seronegative primary to seropositive primary to secondary to late syphilis.

Therefore, it is probable, but unproven, that a longer duration of therapy is required to effect a cure as the infection progresses. For these reasons, the use of more prolonged penicillin therapy, than that recommended by the US public health service when treating secondary or latent syphilis, should be considered.

Q 100

A 20-year-old Buddhist nun from Sikkim is admitted after collapsing at her monastery. She has not been abroad for the last three years. She has no significant history and was apparently well four hours prior to admission.

On examination, she is hypotensive with an unrecordable blood pressure, pulse rate 80/min, regular. JVP is not elevated and the heart-sounds are normal. She is apyrexial and the rest of the examination is unremarkable.

Results:
• Hb – 13.2 g/dl

- WBC – 5.4 x 10^9/L
- Platelets –131x 10^9L
- Sodium – 138 mmols/L
- Potassium – 3.0 mmols/L
- Urea – 4.3 mg/L
- Creatinine – 80 mmol/L
- pH – 7.38
- PO_2 – 10.5 kPa
- PCO_2 – 5.2 kPa
- SaO_2 – 95
- Chest X-ray – normal
- ECG-sinus rhythm – PR interval 0.12 sec, QRS duration 0.4 sec (Wide QRS)

A. WHAT IS THE DIAGNOSIS?

ANS: This patient is suffering from a quinine overdose as a consequence of treatment for cerebral malaria.

Because quinidine is more cardiotoxic than quinine, its administration is cardiologically monitored with full vital signs equipment and with the appropriate interventional drugs on hand if dysrrhythmia and hypertension are to be avoided or terminated.

A blood-level in excess of (7 mg/L) of quinine, an electrographic QT interval more than 55 ms, a QRS prolongation more than 120 ms or a QTc of more than 20% of the baseline is an indication of an overdose. Arrhythmia may develop due to choloquine overdose since it is a negative inotropic agent.

In this case, the blood glucose value should be measured every 4–6 hours. If the blood glucose value drops below 40 mg/dl, the patient should receive intravenous dextrose (0.3 g/kg). All quinine administration should receive a continuous infusion of 5–10% dextrose.

Q 101

A 7-year-old elder son of a security guard, recently relocated to Lahore, developed a sore throat. A local doctor suggested an aspirin gargle, but this did not relieve his discomfort. The physician described exudative pharyngitis and treated him with penicillin. This resulted in prompt recovery. However, two weeks later he has swelling of the face and ankle, and haematuria.

On examination, he is afebrile and his throat appears to be normal. Pulse 96/min, blood pressure 144/96 mmHg. JVP raised 4 cm with bilateral pedal oedema. There is no evidence of heart-failure and the rest of the clinical examination is normal.

- Hb – 10.1 g/dl
- WBC – 5.2 x 10⁹/L
- Platelets – 182 x 10⁹/L
- Sodium – 131 mmol/L
- Potassium – 4.7 mmol/L
- Urea – 13.8 mmol/L
- Creatinine – 271 mmol/L
- ESR – 59 mm/h
- Chest X-ray – normal

A. WHAT IS THE MOST LIKELY DIAGNOSIS?
ANS: This boy has post-streptococcal glomerulonephritis.

The treatment of acute post streptococcal glomerulonephritis is supportive. One should recommend bedrest until the size of the glomerular inflammation and circulatory congestion (primary hypertension) normalise. Prolonged inactivity is of benefit in the healing process. Fluid retention, circulatory congestion and oedema may be treated with sodium, fluid restriction or loop diuretics. Diuresis alone often ameliorates hypertension. If severe hypertension is present, vasodilators such as nitroprusside, nifedipine or hydralise may be useful.

Encephalopathy and pulmonary congestion generally improve with the lowering of the blood pressure and the relieving of the circulatory overload. Digitalis should be avoided, except in well-documented organic heart disease with congestive heart failure. Treatment with ion exchange resin or dialysis may be required for severe oliguria, fluid overload and hyperkalaemia. Mild protein restriction is indicated in azotemic patients. A 7–10 days course of antimicrobial therapy eg. Penicillin or erythromycin should be given if streptococcal infection is documented. Long-term chemoprophylaxis is not indicated. Glucocorticoids and cytotoxic drugs are of no value.

Acute glomerulonephritis following group A Streptococcus is the prototype of the disease that causes acute nephritis. Immune complexes deposit in the subepithelial region of the glomerulocapillary wall, between the basement membrane and the visceral epithelial cell that separates that membrane from the urinary space, and provoke a transient but intense inflammatory process. GFR falls, but returns within weeks to months in most patients. Deposition of immune complexes is also believed to be the cause of acute nephritis, (following other bacteria and viral infections) and lupus nephritis, membranoproliferative glomerulonephritis, Henoch-Schonlein purpura and Buerger's disease, i.e. Ig A nephropathy.

Renal biopsy is usually required for the evaluation of patients with acute nephritis to see whether rapidly aggressive renal failure is present. Rheumatic fever is not a sequel to streptococcal skin infection, in contrast to pharyngitis, although post-streptococcal glomerulonephritis may follow either skin or throat infection. The reason for this difference is not known. One possibility is that the immune response necessary for the development of rheumatic fever only occurs with the infection of the pharyngeal mucosa. In addition, the strain of Group A streptococci that causes pharyngitis are generally of different M-protein types from those causing skin infection, suggesting the strain that causes pharyngitis may have rheumatogenic potential, while the skin strain does not.

Q 102

A 5-year-old boy has had high temperature, persistent at 38°C despite antibiotics, for five days. He develops a rash four days after the onset of fever and complains of pain in his neck and lips.

On examination, he is unwell, irritable and has a temperature of 39.6°C, pulse 120/min irregular, blood pressure 110/ 70 mmHg. Heart sounds are normal with a pansystolic murmur and a third heart sound. Examination of the abdomen, chest and the central nervous system turns up nothing abnormal. He has bilateral cervical lymphadenopathy. His pharynx is red, but there are no ulcers or exudate. His lips are red with cracks and he has a wide spread morbliform rash with reddening of the palms and desquamation of the finger tips.

Investigation:
• Bilateral conjunctival erythaema is noted.

- Hb – 10.3 g/dl
- WBC – 18.3 x 10^9/L
- Platelets – 1,016 x 10^9/L
- ESR – 110 mm
- CRP – 93 mmol/L
- Bilirubin – 8 μmol/L
- AST – 69 IU/L
- ALT – 114 IU/L
- Albumin – 31 g/L
- Chest X-ray – Normal lung fields, but the the size of the heart is at the upper range of normal. ECG shows a sinus rhythm with multiple atrial and ventricular premature beats. There is first degree heart block, widespread non-specific ST- and T-wave changes.

A. What is the diagnosis?
Ans: This patient has Kawasaki's disease and should be treated with a high dosage of aspirin and intravenous gammaglobulins. Enhocardiography should be performed to examine the coronary arteries.

B. What other diagnoses would you consider in this condition?
Ans: Toxic shock syndrome, Rocky Mountain spotted fever, meningococcemia, streptococcal scarlet fever, toxic epidermal necrolysis and a syndrome following Group A streptococcal infection.

Q 103

A 43-year-old woman, who collects meteorites for trade, is admitted with a history of diplopia. She was well until 10 hours ago when she developed dry mouth and a sense that something was wrong. She noticed blurring of the vision and by the time she arrived at the hospital, she was seeing double. She travels extensively in search of rare meteorites. She sustained a wound about 11 days ago when she fell down while searching the site of a reported meteorite fall.

On examination, she appears afebrile, pulse 110/min regular, blood pressure 120/80 mmHg lying and 105/65 mmHg. Her pupils are fixed and dilated, but the fundus is normal. She complains of diplopia in all directions of gaze and the extracular movements of both eyes are impaired. She has dysarthria and reduced gag reflex. Her tongue is normal. There is weakness of shoulder shrugging and abduction bilaterally, but the limb reflexes are normal, although the biceps jerk could only be elicited with the Jendrassic manoeuvre. The rest of the neurological examinations are normal, though she has a palpable bladder. She has a deep gash, bandaged, in her left shin.

- Hb – 13.1 g/dl
- WBC – 6.4 x 10⁹/L
- Platelets – 361 x 10⁹/L
- Sodium – 143 mmol/L
- Potassium – 4.9 mmol/L
- Urea – 4.3 mmol/L
- Creatinine – 78 µmol/L
- Examination of the CSF – normal
- ECG – a sinus rhythm with non-specific ST- and T-wave changes.
- Lung function test – a restrictive pattern
- Tensilon test – normal

A. WHAT IS THE LIKELY DIAGNOSIS?
ANS: This patient has wound botulism.

When wounds are contaminated with clostridium botinum spores, the spores germinate into a vegetative organism that produces toxin. This condition resembles a blood-borne illness, except that the incubation period averages about 10 days and gastrointestinal symptoms are absent. Wound botulism has been noted after traumatic wounds are contaminated by soil, in drug abusers and after a caesarean section. The wound may appear benign.

The demonstration of toxins in serum bioassay in mice is definitive, but the test may be negative, particularly in wound and infant botulism. It is only performed by specific laboratories that can be identified by contacting regional public health authorities. The presence of the toxins or organisms in the vomitus, gastric fluid or stool is highly suggestive, because intestinal carriage is rare. Wound cultures showing the organisms are suggestive. The edrophonium chloride (Tensilon test) for myasthenia gravis may be mildly positive in botulism, but is usually less dramatic.

In wound botulism, equine antitoxin is administered. The wound should be thoroughly explored and debrided and an antibiotic such as penicillin should be given to eradicate *clostridium botulinum*, although the benefit of this therapy is unproven. The results of the wound culture should be used to guide the use of other antibiotics.

Type A disease is more severe than type B and the mortality is higher above the age of 60. Artificial respiratory support may be required in severe cases. Some patients experience weakness and autonomic dysfunction for as long as one year after the disease's onset. Although botulinum toxin is lethal in high doses, it is used in a highly diluted form as therapy for strabismus, cosmetic treatment, blepharospasm and other dystonias in advanced neurological centres. In patients with botulism, the response to repetitive stimulation is similar to that of the Eaton-Lambert syndrome, although the findings are variable and not all muscles are affected.

Q 104

A 34-year-old navy aviator, a pilot on a VTOL carrier, has a 2-week history of dry cough, breathlessness and inability to take deep breaths. He has flown several combat missions and served with distinction during the recent Middle East conflict.

On examination, he is febrile. Temperature 37.9°C. The examination reveals a tattoo of his combat division on the right shoulder, acquired while posted in Subic Bay. He was a flight instructor in Manila eight years ago. He denies any drug abuse and recently got married to a screen writer. This patient has seborrheic dermatitis.

Investigation:
- Hb – 13.2 g/dl
- WBC – 4.2 x 10/L
- Platelets – 425 x 10/L
- Serum LDH – elevated
- Chest X-ray – A possible interstitial shadowing around the right hilum. A day after the chest X-ray was taken, he developed pneumothorax which was treated.

A. What is the most likely diagnosis?

Ans: HIV acquired through unsterile tattoo equipment. Predisposing to Pneumocystis Carinii Pneumonia (PCP). Approximately 70–80% of patients with HIV infection will experience, at least once, PCP some time during the course of the disease and PCP is listed as the immediate cause of death for up to 20% of patients with AIDS. The risk of infection by pneumocystic carinii increases when the CD4 + T cell-count declines. Patients with HIV are most likely to experience PCP when the CD4 + T cell count falls below 200/microlitre. The usual clinical findings of pneumonia are not present. Breathe sounds are usually clear, possibly slightly diminished. PCP is complicated by pneumothorax in approximately 2% of cases.

The patient should undergo HIV testing after appropriate sympathetic counseling by an expert. He should be induced to produce sputum and a bronchioalveolar lavage should be performed. The fluid should be Groccot-stained (silver stain) to demonstrate the trophozoite or cyst forms of the organism. (PCR has been used in attempts to identify specific DNA sequences for pneumocystic carinii in clinical specimens.) Blood should be taken for culture and sensitivity. An arterial blood gas should be performed at rest and repeated after exercise to look for desaturation.

The mortality for patients with PCP associated with pneumothorax is approximately 10% and aggressive medical (sclerotherapy) and surgical intervention may be required. Pneumocystic carinii is capable of haematogenous spread and may seed a variety of organ systems, as well cause a primary infection of the ear. Pneumocystic carinii may also cause a necrotising vasculitis that resembles Buerger's disease, bone marrow hypoplasia and intestinal obstruction.

PCP may be treated with trimethoprim/sulphamethoxazole, effective in nine out of 10 patients. Up to 50% of the HIV population treated with this drug developed side effects such as rash, fever, leucopenia, thrombocytopenia and hepatitis. Therapy need not be stopped when this occurs. It is important to remain vigilant for more serious hypersensitivity reactions such as the Stevens-Johnson syndrome.

It is now mild malpractice not to treat a HIV patient with a combination of triple drug anti-viral chemotherapeutic regime, one of which must be a protease inhibitor. Paradoxically during the first five days of treatment of PCP, there may be a worsening of the patient's condition secondary to the inflammatory response, resulting from a large number of organisms in the lungs. This inflammatory response can be attenuated by the use of glucocorticoids. Glucocorticoids can also reduce thickening at the alveolar capillary interface. Although this appears counterintuitive in an already immunosuppressed patient, the only significant side effect is an increased incidence of thrush.

Anaphylaxis is extremely rare in patients with HIV infection. Patients, with cutaneous eruptions during a single course of therapy, can still be considered candidates for further treatment and prophylaxis with the same agent.

Q 105

A 26-year-old sales representative for a major drug company has been treated for pneumocystic carinii. He recovers and has refused an HIV test. He has lost a great deal of weight during the last six months. He travels widely and was admitted to a missionary hospital for treatment of suspected malaria as the area he was traversing was endemic with this disease.

On examination, he has seborrheic dermatitis and fundoscopy reveals some cotton wool-like spots.

Results:
• Blood film – No malarial parasites, but there is thrombocytopenia.
• APTT – 73 seconds (control 41 seconds)
• PT – 14 seconds (control 15 seconds)

A. WHAT IS THE EXPLANATION FOR HIS HAEMATOLOGICAL INDICES?
ANS: The APTT is prolonged due to the lupus anticoagulant which has been reported in patients with AIDS. The lupus anticoagulants belongs to the family of anti-phospholipid antibodies. It is recognised by the prolongation of partial thromboplasma time and failure of added plasma to correct the prolongation.

More sensitive tests include the Russell fibre venom time and the rabbit brain neutrophospholipid test. Antibodies to cardiolipin are detected in ELISA assays. Clinical manifestations of lupus anticoagulant and antibodies to cardiolipin include thrombocytopenia, recurrent venous or arterial clotting, recurrent foetal loss and valvular heart disease.

If the lupus anticoagulant is associated with hypoprothrombinaemia or thrombocytopenia, bleeding may develop. Less commonly, antibodies to clotting factors VIII and IX develop, causing bleeding. The bleeding syndrome usually responds to glucocorticoids; clotting syndromes do not. The lupus anticoagulant is therefore an in vitro anticoagulant, but an in vivo coagulant. Lupus anticoagulants are seen most commonly in patients with SLE, but they are also seen in association with other collagen vascular diseases.

Circulation of anticardiolipin antibodies (lupus anticoagulant) is associated with strokes in young adults, although its relative frequency is controversial.

Q 106

A 35-year-old carpenter was diagnosed as having AIDS four years ago. He had oesophageal candiadiasis and was found to be HIV positive. He was treated successfully for pneumocystic carinii pneumonia nine months ago. He was on zidovudine QDS and protease inhibitor for the first one and half years following the diagnosis of AIDS, but he developed bone marrow depression and the dosage of zidovudine was reduced to its current 250 mg. He has been taking nebulised pentamidine as PCP prophylaxis. He gives a 4-month history of increasing malaise, night sweats and diarrhoea. There is no headache. He has no neurological symptoms. He has not travelled outside England.

On examination, he is febrile with a temperature of 38.3°C and has lost a great deal of weight.

Results:
- Hb – 9.8 g/d1
- WBC – 3.1 x 10^9 /L
- Platelets – 146 x 10^9/L
- Sodium – 138 mmol/L
- Potassium – 3.6 mmol/L
- Urea – 5.1 mmol/L
- Creatinine – 97 µmol/L
- Bilirubin – 13 mmol/L
- AST – 65 IU/L
- ALT – 197 IU/L
- Albumin – 33 g/L
- SaO$_2$ – 98% on air
- Chest X-ray – Normal
- Stool cultures – No significant growth

- Colonoscopic examination – A neoplasm in the colon. Histopathology proves this to be intestinal lymphoma.
- Blood culture and sensitivity – Negative.

A.WHAT IS THE MOST LIKELY DIAGNOSIS?

ANS: This patient has atypical tuberculosis. This patient has mycobacterium avium complex (MAC).

This group of organisms may be referred to collectively as *mycobacterium intracellularae* (MAI). Now commercially available specific nucleic acid probes provide rapid and convenient differentiation of *mycobacterium avium* and *mycobacterium intracellularae*. When the lungs are involved, the clinical pictures frequently mimic pulmonary tuberculosis. The patient may show lower zone nodular subpleural shadowing, bronchiectasis or a solitary nodule.

When a MAC organism is isolated from a patient with pulmonary disease, it is important to be certain of the pathogeny of the organism in the disease because chemotherapy is often associated with morbidity. The most important risk factor appears to be CD4 count of 100 cells x 10^6/L of blood. Involvement of the small intestine may produce watery diarrhoea and malabsorption.

The finding of hepatosplenomagaly, thickening of the small bowel wall and lymphodepathy in the abdominal CT scan suggest MAC infection. The diagnosis of disseminated MAC infection is made by isolation of organisms from the blood, bone marrow or liver tissues. Radiomatching blood culture system can quickly confirm the diagnosis in disseminated diseases, and nucleic acid probes can facilitate rapid species identification. The usual survival rate is only 4–10 months once the diagnosis of disseminated MAC infection has been made, but therapy reduces morbidity in some patients and may extend survival.

Strains of mycobacterium avium in patients with AIDS are more likely to be from Serovars one and eight and produce pigments containing plasmids and have a particular RFLP (Restriction Fragment Length Polymorphism) pattern. Treatment of MAC infections is difficult and often unsatisfactory. The organisms are often resistant to most conventional anti-mycobacterium drugs. Mild diabetes insipidus may worsen or improve during pregnancy. AVP-resistant diabetes insipidus may also develop during pregnancy, perhaps due to increased circulating levels of placental vasopressinase. Fortunately, such patients respond to treatment with desmopressin.

B. WHAT ARE THE MOST IMPORTANT INVESTIGATIONS?

ANS:

i)   Cortisol level

ii) Thyroid function test

iii) LH-SH/ oestradiol

iv) Combined pituitary stimulation test.

Blood samples have been taken from patients A, B and C for the Paul-Bunnell test.

PATIENT	NO ABSORPTION	GUINEA PIG ABSORPTION	OX RED CELL ABSORPTION
A	+	+	-
B	+	-	+
C	+	-	-

A. WHAT IS THE LIKELY DIAGNOSIS FOR EACH PATIENT?

ANS:

Patient A has infectious mononucleosis.

Patient B has a false antibody (which may be normal or suggests lymphoma).

Patient C has serum sickness.

B. WHAT ARE HETEROPHILE ANTIBODIES?

ANS: These are antibodies to sheep erythrocytes, which can be removed by prior absorption with beef red blood cells, but not with guinea pig kidneys. These are demonstrated in 50% of children and 90–95% of adults with mononucleosis.

   Although the classic heterophile titre is performed in many laboratories, the Monospot test using a commercial kit sensitive titre is routinely employed to diagnose mononucleosis. The frequency of heterophil positivity associated with infectious mononucleosis depends upon the test used and can also be affected by the age of the patient and the phase of the illness when the test is administered. The Monospot test may be slightly more sensitive than the heterophile titres.

   Ten to 15 percent of patients with mononucleosis may be heterophil negative. This is particularly true if they are tested during the first week of the illness before an antibody response can be mounted. If clinical suspicion of monocleosis is high, testing of heterophile antibodies during the second or third week of the illness is necessary. Heterophile antibodies decline in titre after the acute illness is resolved, but may be detected up to nine months after the onset of the illness.

Q 108

A 23-year-old pianist, studying at the Royal Academy of Music, collapses outside her student hall one day. She has been working part-time as an auxillary nurse for the last six months. On admission into the hospital, her blood glucose is 1.7 mmols/L

A. WHAT OTHER TESTS WOULD YOU PERFORM TO INVESTIGATE THE CAUSE OF HER HYPOGLYCAEMIA?
ANS: I would test for insulin levels with a simultaneous C peptide assay. The C peptide would not be present in the presence of synthetic insulin, whereas an elevation in C peptide without a correlated elevation in insulin suggests factitious hypoglycaemia.
   I would also test for sulfonylurea in the urine.

Q 109

A 34-year-old diplomat suffers increasing pain when he sneezes. He has a recent history of loin pain. He sweats excessively and has had severe headaches for six months.

Investigation:
- Serum calcium – 2.5 mmols/L
- Serum phosphate – 1.2 mmols/L
- Albumin – 40 g/L
- Urine calcium – 11 mmols/L (less than seven is normal)
- Fasting glucose – 12 mmols/L
- X-ray of the knee joints – Evidence of calcium pyrophosphate deposition.

A. What is the diagnosis?

Ans: This patient has acromegaly.

This may be associated with calcium pyrophosphate deposition. Hypercalcuria and a net negative calcium balance occur in acromegaly. Occasionally, osteoporosis is present. Secondary panhypopituitarism and the associated gonadal insufficiency may be a factor in the production of osteoporosis.

Two screening tests available are measurement of glucose suppressed growth hormone concentration and IGF-1/SM-C concentration. The growth hormone concentrations are measured 1–2 hours after the oral administrations of 100 g of glucose. Although a serum growth hormone concentration of less than 5 micrograms/L has traditionally been accepted as normal, a post-suppression value of less than 2 microgram/L is a more rigorous criterion and should be applied. Acromegalics usually have a growth hormone concentration after glucose administration of more than 10. Some acromegalics may suppress below five, but rarely below two micrograms/L. IGF-1/SM-C concentration provides an excellent screening test for acromegaly.

All patients with large pituitary adenomas should be screened with growth hormone measurements, preferably after glucose ingestion. In rare cases, patients with elevated serum growth hormones and IGF-1SM-C concentration may have large pituitary tumours without evidence of acromegaly. This syndrome is unexplained. A majority of patients with acromegaly and most men with prolactinomas have macroadenomas at the time of diagnosis.

B. How would you confirm the diagnosis?

Ans: One may perform an oral glucose tolerance test where there is failure to suppress growth hormone. One can also perform a CT scan of pituitary fossa or an MRI.

Basal or random growth hormone estimation may be supressed in normal people, particularly in women, and in people with uncontrolled diabetes mellitus and renal failure or stress. Therefore, random growth hormone estimation should not be used to screen for acromegaly.

C. How would you treat the patient?

Ans: The patient can be treated with Yttrium implants (an invasive procedure) or medically with bromocryptine or somastatin.

Q110

An 18-year-old hotel manager has numbness of both legs. He has had problems joining in games and appears to be unable to keep up with his friends while walking.

Results of nerve conduction studies:
- Sural nerve action potential – 1 mV (usually more than 4 mV)
- Median nerve action potential – 3 mV (usually more than 10 mV)
- Common peroneal conduction velocity – 50 m/sec (usually more than 40 m/sec)
- Prominent fibrillation potential, fasciculations and high amplitude long duration polyhasic motor potential are seen.

A. WHAT IS THE DIAGNOSIS?
ANS: This patient has hereditary sensory and motor neuropathy type II.

Q 111

A 20-year-old lumberjack has enlargement of his neck nodes, fever and dysarthria. He has been having intermittent fever for the last three months. He smokes occasionally, but does not drink alchohol.

On examination, he has a non-tender cervical lymphadenopathy and is dysarthric with nystagmus in all directions of gaze. He is unsteady on his legs and has been suspended from using a power-saw. The finger-nose test and the heel-shin test show of loss of motor control. He has an extremely unsteady broad-based gait. The Romberg's sign is negative. The unsteadiness does not increase when he closes his eyes. His Mantoux test is negative. Over the next few weeks, the patient develops bladder incontinence and some sensory loss in the legs.

A. WHAT IS THE DIAGNOSIS?
ANS: This patient has cerebellar degeneration, secondary to lymphoma and necrotising myelopathy.

Necrotising myelopathy is a rare complication of lymphoma presenting as subacute transverse myelitis, often in a thoracic zone. It can be distinguished from a less fulminant encephalomyelitis by the evolution of an intensely necrotic cord lesion which tails off caudally and rostrally over several segments. There are multiple necrotic foci within the cord. Clinical findings include weakness and sensory loss of the arms and legs in, initially, an asymmetrical manner mimicking the Brown-Sequard syndrome.

There may be urinary bladder and sphincter abnormalities as in the patient above. In severe cases of necrotising myelopathy, the CSF protein and cell counts are increased, and myelography shows focal cord swellings. Necrotising myelopathy may also be associated with bronchogenic carcinoma and leukaemia.

Q 112

A 54-year-old barrister has had intermittent problems of chewing and swallowing for the last five months. Over the last year, she has lost a great deal of weight and suffered from episodes of diarrhoea. She feels lethargic and had found it increasingly difficult to defend her clients in court as her voice would weaken or change character in the middle of a cross-examination. Some of her colleagues were worried she was under a great deal of stress and may be in the midst of a nervous breakdown. Three months ago she noticed she had difficulty climbing stairs and subsequently had nasal regurgitation of fluids. She has no relevant history, except an episode of syphilis for which she was adequately treated and she underwent an endoscopic examination for erosive gastritis six years ago. Her colleagues had noticed she was increasingly short-tempered, worried and uncharacteristically rude to many of her clients and partners.

On examination, her pulse is 110/min regular, BP 120/70 mmHg and the rest of her physical examination is normal. She has a mild weakness of neck flexion, but the cranial nerves are normal. She is unable to stand from a squatting position. There is weakness and tender muscles of all limbs. Reflexes are normal and the plantars are down going.

Results:
- Sodium – 136 mmol /L
- Potassium – 4.6 mmols/L
- Urea – 5.9 mmol/L
- Creatinine – 105 µmol/L
- Bilirubin – 10 µmol/L

- AST – 43 IU/L
- ALT – 140 IU/L
- CK – 410 IU/L
- Hb – 14.1 g/dl
- WBC – 7.9 x 10^9/L
- Platelets – 346 x 10^9/L

A. WHAT ARE THE TWO DIAGNOSES THAT, IN COMBINATION, WOULD ACCOUNT FOR HER SYMPTOMS?
ANS: Myasthenia gravis and thyrotoxicosis.

Q 113

A 36-year-old army commando, recently returned from a mission in the swamplands of Papua New Guinea, has a 3-day history of irratibility and restlessness.

On examination, he is febrile with pursing of the lips, contraction of the orbicularis oculi and a stiff neck. The musculature of the trunks and limbs are rigid, but the tendon reflexes are retained and he is lucid. He has not been on any phenothiazines. There are multiple minor cuts in his lower limbs for which he has been treated with sulphadiazine cream.

A. WHAT IS THE DIAGNOSIS?
ANS: This patient has tetanus.

Tennis racket or drumstick spores may survive for years in some environments and are resistant to disinfectants and boiling for 20 minutes. Vegetative cells, however, are easily inactivated and are susceptible to antibiotics such as penicillin. Tetanus, notably in the form of skin pulping, has also been associated with burns, frost-bite, ear infection, surgery, abortion, childbirth, and drug abuse.

Autonomic dysfunction may complicate the clinical scenario with tachycardia, hyperpyrexia, arrhythmias, profuse sweating, peripheral vasoconstriction and increased plasma urinary catecholamine levels. Pacemaker insertion is, occasionally, required. Sudden cardiac arrest may occur, but the basis for this is unknown. Complications to be expected are pneumonia, fractures, muscle rupture, deep vein thrombosis, phlebitis, pulmonary embolism, decubitus ulcer and rhabdomyolysis.

Local tetanus is an uncommon form in which manifestations are restricted to muscles near the wound. The prognosis for this unique form of tetanus is excellent. The diagnosis of tetanus is made entirely on the basis of clinical findings.

B. What different diagnosis would you consider?
Ans: Strychnine poisoning, dystonic drug reactions, eg. Phenothiazines and metachlorpromide, hypocalcemic tetany, meningoencephalitis, rabies and trismus may be caused by conditions such as an alveolar abscess.

The marked increased tone in central muscles (face, neck, back, chest and abdomen), with superimposed generalised spasms and relative sparing of the hands and feet, strongly suggests tetanus.

C. What are the goals of therapy?
Ans: They are to eliminate the source of toxin, neutralise the unbound toxin, prevent muscle spasm and provide respiratory support until recovery.

The patient should be admitted to a quiet room in an ICU where observation and cardiac monitoring can be maintained continuously, but stimulation is minimal. Protection of the airway is critical. Wounds should be explored carefully and thoroughly debrided. Parenteral penicillin (10–12 million units daily x 10 days) could be administered to eradicate vegetative cells, the source of the toxin, although it is of unknown value. Clindamycin, erythromycin and metronidazole may be given as substitutes for patients with penicillin allergy.

Active immunisation should be initiated because immunity is not induced by a small amount of toxin that produces the disease. Active immunisation should, therefore, be paradoxically initiated. The patient should be adequately hydrated, given adequate enteral or parenteral nutrition, and physiotherapy should be performed to prevent contractures. Heparin should be given to prevent pulmonary embolism. Gastrointestinal bleeding and decubitus ulcer must be prevented and intercurrent infection should be treated. The course of tetanus extends for up to six weeks and patients may require ventilatory support for three weeks during this period. Increased tone and minor spasms can last for months, but recovery is usually complete.

Q 114

A 26-year-old nun, serving in a South American tribal community, has a 2-day history of occipital headache, photophobia and vomiting. She collapsed while attempting to preach.

On examination, she is febrile with a temperature of 39.3°C. There is neck stiffness and a fundoscopy reveals bilateral papilloedema. The neurological examination does not reveal any significant findings and the plantars are both downgoing. An abdominal examination does not reveal any visceromegaly. A thick and thin smear for malarial parasite (endemic in that area) is negative. On being transported by helicopter to the nearest hospital, she is subjected to a lumbar puncture.

Findings:
- Opening pressure – 18 cm H_2O
- Red cell – 2/mm^3
- White cell – 240 (80% lymphocytes)
- Protein – 0.51 g/L
- Glucose – 3.3 mmol/l
- Blood level – 5.2 mmol/l

She was treated with morphine and an antiemetic. Her symptoms improved over the next few days. However, the headache recurred the following day and was worsened by any movement. She became drowsy and had five seizures involving the right leg.

A. WHAT IS THE DIAGNOSIS?
ANS: This patient has thrombosis of the sagittal sinus which is predisposed by viral meningitis with recurrent vomiting and dehydration.

The diagnosis is readily made by magnetic resonance angiography, intravenous digital subtraction angiography. The coagulation indices of this patient should be performed. The urea and electrolytes status should be analysed. She should be adequately hydrated, anticoagulated with intravenous heparin and started on a loading dose of phenytoin.

Q 115

A 74-year-old ex-SAS major has noticed a progressive weakness of his left hand with a wasting of small muscles over a period of eight months. He has a long history of neck and shoulder pain, but feels this is due to past injuries in combat. He has an occasional occipital headache, but otherwise he leads a healthy lifestyle. He has no symptoms in his right arm or lower limbs. He has noticed mild urinary frequency and nocturia for the last four months, but was reassured by some of his colleagues that it was probably just prostatism, common in a man of his age.

He used to smoke a pipe, but gave up the habit about six months ago. During bouts of coughing and sneezing, the patient does not appreciate any radiating pain in his arm or shoulder. There is nothing in his medical history suggestive of any whiplash injury to the spine. He takes no medication, but confesses he used to be on amphetamines during training when he was much younger.

On examination, there is a restriction in lateral rotatory movement in his neck. The cranial nerves are normal. There is wasting of the small muscles of his left hand and left forearm and there is weakness in finger extension, finger abduction and thumb abduction on the left side. On the right, mild weakness on finger extension was noted. Lower limb reflexes and sensation are normal. No fasciculation is seen. He had a hyperinflated chest with scattered expiratory wheeze, but is otherwise well.

Results of the initial investigation are as follows:
- Cervical spine X-ray. There is no intervebral narrowing and no subluxation. There is no reversal of the normal cervical curvature and there is no reduction of the sagittal diameter of the canal even with neck extension. There is no spondylotic bar formed by osteophytes arising from the dorsal surface of adjacent vertebral bodies. The absence of this suggests there is no radiological evidence of a horizontal compression of the ventral cord.
- Chest X-ray – no abnormality apart from hyperinflation and there are no cervical ribs present
- CT scan and MRI of the neck revealed an absence of cervical cord compression. There is no evidence of disc rupture.
- Electromyography does not demonstrate radicular compression.
- CT myelogram does not show any evidence suggestive of cervical disc disease nor any evidence of spondolytic compressive myelopathy or radiculopathy. There is no narrowing of the neural foramen.
- Serum B 12 – normal

A. WHAT IS THE DIAGNOSIS WHICH WOULD EXPLAIN THIS PATIENT'S CLINICAL PICTURE?

ANS: Motor neuron disease.

Cervical spondylosis is both an under and overdiagnosed disease. Although radiographic findings of spondylosis are common in the elderly, only a few patients develop myelopathy or radiculopathy, often dependant on a congenitally narrow canal. Many patients with intrinsic cord process, particularly amyotropic lateral sclerosis, multiple selerosis and subacute combined degeneration, have undergone cervical laminectomies in the belief that spondylosis was responsible.

There may be temporary improvement suggesting there is an element of spondylotic compression, but the underlying intrinsic myelopathy soon progresses.

The safety of the new water soluble ionic contrast material has made myelography a more feasible procedure associated with less risk. The obsolete iodophendylate myelography should not be confused with this. Furthermore, residual iodophendylate after myelography produces artifacts on subsequent MRI scans.

In motor neuron disease, EMG will show denervation changes in the muscle of both the upper and lower limbs including the clinically uninvolved muscles.

Q 116

A 42-year-old architect has an 8-week history of seeing double, numbness of the left side of the face and a sense of unsteadiness. He usually visits construction sites, but no longer does so for fear of falling off beams. For the last 10 days he has been depressed, fearing he has lost his creativity and his ability to conceptualise forms in three dimensions. Three years ago he had developed a bilateral 7th nerve palsy which recovered completely after a course of steroids.

On examination, he sees double on horizontal gaze and says the images are seen side by side (horizontal diplopia). There is decreased sensation to pin-pricks and cold over the left side of his face, absent abduction of the left eye, and left sided motor neuron facial weakness. His eyes have small yellow nodules visible on the conjunctiva. His gait is unsteady with a tendency to deviate towards the left. There was past-pointing and dysdiadochokinesia on the right. An abdominal examination reveals a 2 cm hepatomegaly and the tip of the spleen is palpable. The cranial CT scan is normal.

Investigation:
- CSF opening pressure – 16 cm H_2O
- Red cells – less than 2/mm^3
- White cells – less than 2/mm^3
- Protein – 1.4 g/L
- Glucose – 3.5 g/L
- Gram stain and Ziehl-Neelsen stain – negative
- Blood glucose – 6 mmol/L

A. WHAT IS THE DIAGNOSIS?

ANS: This patient has neurosarcoidosis.

Sarcoidosis is a chronic multisystem of phagocytes, non-caseating epitheloid granulomas and derangement of the normal tissue architecture in affected organs. All parts of the body can be affected by sarcoidosis. Thus, it may be confused with many other disorders. Therefore, different diagnoses should always be considered.

Neurological involvement occurs in 5% of patients. The most common is 7th nerve involvement with unilateral facial palsy. It occurs suddenly and is usually temporary. Other common manifestations of neurosarcoidosis include optic nerve dysfunction, papilloedema, palate dysfunction, hearing abnormalities, hypothalamic and pituitary abnormalities, chronic meningitis and space-occupying lesion.

Psychiatric manifestations have been described and seizures can occur. It is rare, but multiple lesions can occur which mimics multiple sclerosis, spinal cord abnormalities and peripheral neuropathics. This diagnosis may be confirmed by MRI with gadolinium enhancement. A CSF ACE level should also be performed.

A liver biopsy would show sarcoid granulomas in the periportal areas. Usually the changes reflect a cholestatic pattern in liver dysfunction, including an elevated alkaline phophatase level; the bilirubin and aminotranferases are only mildly elevated and jaundice is rare. Rarely, portal hypertension can occur as an intrahepatic cholestasis with cirrhosis.

Autopsy shows that sarcoidosis involves most organs in a majority of patients, but the disease manifests clinically only in organs where it affects function. Although splenomegaly occurs in only 5–10% of patients, coeliac angiography or splenic biopsy reveals involvement in 50–60% of cases of sarcoidosis.

The presence of skin allergy is not diagnostic of sarcoidosis. The Kveim-Siltzbach skin test, an intradermal injection of a heat-treated suspension of sarcoidosis spleen extract, when biopsied 4–6 weeks later yields sarcoid-like lesions in 70–80% of individuals with sarcoidosis, with less than 5% false positive results. The material is not widely available and there is controversy in regards to its use as a diagnostic tool.

Although no blood findings are diagnostic of sarcoidosis, the serum angiotensin converting enzyme is elevated in approximately 2/3 of patients with sarcoidosis, but false positive and false negative results are common. The chest X-ray may support sarcoidosis with a finding of bilateral hilar lymphadenopathy.

Biopsy evidence of mononuclear cell granulamatous inflammatory process is necessary in order to make a definitive diagnosis of sarcoidosis. The histological picture is not sufficient to make the diagnosis since non-caseating granulomas are found in other diseases including infections and malignancies.

B. How would you treat this patient?

Ans: The therapy of choice is glucocorticoids.

Other drugs such as indomethacin, oxyphenbutazone, chloroquine, methotrexate, p-amino benzoate, allopurinal, levamisole and cyclophosphamides have been used, but there has been no randomised double blind control trial apart from anecdotal reports to support their beneficial effects.

Cyclosporin is not effective for the pulmonary manifestations of sarcoidosis, but anecdotal evidence suggest that it may be used for extrathoracic sarcoidosis not responding to glucorticoids.

The disease clears spontaneously in 50% of patients and permanent organ derangement often do not improve with steroids. The usual regime is prednisolone 1 mg/kg x 4–6 weeks, followed by a slow tapering over 2–3 months. This is repeated if the disease becomes active again. Inhaled glucocorticoids are not effective.

Q 117

A 42-year-old pilot is admitted with a 3-day history of fever and drowsiness. He is dysarrthric and unable to stand unsupported. Six weeks ago, in Hong Kong, he had eaten an exotic Chinese preparation comprising steamed pork tongues.

The cranial CT scan is normal.

The CSF findings:
- Opening pressure – 24 cm H_2O
- Red cell – less than 2/mm^3
- White cells – 90 (75% polymorphs)/mm^3
- Protein – 0.84 g/dl
- Glucose – 2.3 mmol/l
- Blood glucose – 6.7 mmol/l

A. WHAT IS THE MOST LIKELY DIAGNOSIS?

ANS: This patient had meningitis due to listeria monocytogenes from contaminated pork tongue. The incubation varies from as early as two weeks to six weeks.

The largest outbreak in the United States occurred in 1985 in Los Angeles. In this outbreak, over 100 cases were reported leading to 48 deaths and still-births. Although food borne transmission appears to the major cause for epidemics and sporadic disease, several clusters of late neonatal onset of the disease suggest nosocomial transmission of listeria monocytogens can occur. Contaminated medical material and equipment has been suggested as the cause for some nosocomial infection.

Listeriosis is an occupational hazard for veterinarians and others who have close contact with infected animals. CSF cultures may be sterile and blood cultures are usually diagnostic. Listeriosis is diagnosed when the organism is cultured from usually sterile sites such as blood, CSF or amniotic fluid. The organism will grow rapidly within 36 hours on routine culture media and cold enrichment may increase the yield.

There are morphological similarities between listeria and both diphtheroids and streptococci. Biochemical tests are required to identify the species. A culture of the organism from non-sterile sites such as the vagina and rectum is not useful for the diagnosis because the organism may be carried in 5% of healthy individuals.

B. How would you treat these patients?
Ans: The treatment of choice is intravenous therapy with ampicillin, often in combination with an aminoglycoside. If the person is allergic to penicillin, trimethoprim sulphamethosazole may be used successfully.

Listeria monocytogenes is susceptible, in vitro, to Penicillin G, erythromycin, ampicillin, trimethoprim-sulphamethosazole, chloramphenicol, rifampicin, tetracyclines, aminoglycosides and imipenern, Chloramphenicol and rifampin may antagonise the antibactericidal effect of penicillin. Cephalosporins are not recommended.

Q 118

A Thai neonatologist with AIDS has a 2-month history of clumsiness and difficulty in climbing stairs and is currently on AZT, a protease inhibitor, and other antiviral drugs, as well as multivitamins. She caught the virus while working in Zambia. During a bloody caesarean section the floor was flooded with blood. She was wearing slippers which unfortunately exposed the wound of a freshly removed ingrown toenail due to infection. She nearly dropped a newborn several days ago. She has lost a great deal of weight and complains of general malaise. Her medical Director had been informed of her medical condition and she has been allowed to continue her medical practice.

On examination, she has wasting of the proximal muscles and weakness. The muscles are not tender and there is no rash.

Results:
- Sodium – 135 mmol/L
- Potassium – 4.4 mmol/L
- Urea – 3.1 mmol/L
- Creatinine – 85 µmol/L
- Thyroid function – normal.
- CK – 1,128 IU/L
- ANA – negative

A. WHAT ARE THE TWO MAIN POSSIBLE DIAGNOSES IN THIS CASE?

ANS: She may either be having HIV associated myopathy or myopathy as a complication of AZT therapy.

Most patients with AZT myopathy have been on therapy for at least six months or more and often have a higher enzyme level and more pain than non-AZT cases. Biopsy is helpful in determining the distinction since AZT related cases show more muscle fibre necrosis and less inflammation than patients with HIV myopathy. Discontinuation of AZT results in a resolution of symptoms in those caused by the drug. Concurrent glucocorticoid therapy may allow continuation of AZT therapy.

The biopsy of HIV myopathy is characterised by inflammation and myofibre degeneration and necrosis.

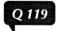

Q 119

A 28-year-old Hong Kong police officer has a 3-day history of fever, confusion and a left-sided weakness. He has been seeing visions of criminals whom he sent to the gallows. He appears to be drowsy, confused, with a mild left-sided weakness and an extensor plantar response on the left. There is no neck stiffness and a CT scan of the skull shows nothing unusual.

Results of the CSF examination:
- Red cells – 210/mm³
- White cells – 120 (85% lymphocytes)/mm³
- Protein – 1.0 g/L
- Glucose – 2.3 mmols/L
- Blood glucose – 5.8 mmols/L
- Gram stain – No organisms seen
- Ziehl-Neelsen – No AFB seen

A. WHAT IS THE MOST LIKELY DIAGNOSIS?

ANS: This patient has Herpes simplex encephalitis and he should be immediately treated with Acyclovir. The patient should be started with intravenous Acyclovir. Nucleotide amplification of viral specific DNA for Herpes simplex virus, using polymerase chain reaction (PCR), may be used as a diagnostic tool to confirm the diagnosis.

Localising signs, hemiplegia, oculogyric crisis and bloody CSF favour the diagnosis of Type 1 Herpes simplex encephalitis (acute haemorrhagic leucoencephalitis). Cisternal and lateral cervical punctures (C1-C2) are safe procedures in the hands of an expert. It is sometimes necessary in instances of spinal block to perform myelography above a lesion. An EEG showing focal or lateralised periodic slow wave complexes, sometimes with a sharpened outline in patients with acute encephalopathy, strongly suggests a diagnosis of herpes simplex encephalitis.

Q 120

A 35-year-old computer programmer has myoclonus and progressive deterioration in the quality of his work. The recent programme he wrote had innumerable mistakes and there appears to be a steady deterioration in the quality of his thought processes as evident in the mistakes in his work. He has no previous medical problem, except for an operation on his eyes – the cornea had been scarred in an accidental exposure to ammonia. He begins to behave in an uncharacteristic manner towards his friends and appears to becoming reclusive. Several days ago, in a fit of anger and for no apparent reason, he smashed his computer screen and walked out of the office.

CSF examination does not show any abnormality, except for a mildly elevated protein level and EEG-demonstrated periodic high amplitude biphasic sharp waves. The full blood count and biochemical profile are normal. Serum B12 and red-cell folate are normal. VDRL and HIV serology are negative.

A. WHAT IS THE DIAGNOSIS?
ANS: This patient has subacute encephalopathy (Creutzfeldt-Jakob disease), a rare dementia transmitted by corneal transplantation.

It is caused by a novel agent known as Prion protein and transmitted by neuro-surgical instrumentation, injection of growth hormones extracted from human pituitaries. In most cases, the route of infection is unknown. After incubation for several years, the illness appears in late life and progresses to death within months. The dementia is often combined with ataxia, cortico-spinal signs, abnormal movements, blindness and myoclonus. Bizarre behaviour and hallucinations are sometimes striking.

In contrast to most infections of the nervous system, signs of intracranial inflammation are absent and CSF is normal, but characteristic EEG abnormality (repetitive complexes) supports the diagnosis. A rare genetic disorder, Gerstmann-Schenker-Strausler disease, is caused by mutation in the prion protein.

Creutzfeldt-Jakob Disease is not contagious, but person to person spread of disease has occurred following transplantation of corneal grafts obtained from infected patients, as well as the use of human cadaver-derived growth hormone and gonadotrophin. Isolated cases have been attributed to improper sterilisation of neurosurgical instruments and stereotactic-intracerebral depth electrodes application. Synthetic growth hormone was developed in 1985, solving the danger of contamination through this supply route.

Myoclonic jerks are noted in more than 90% of patients and can be provoked by a startle stimuli such as surprise or shock. Two-thirds of infected patients will develop Parkinsonian extrapyramidal symptoms with hypokinesis. The clinical dementia appears disproportionate to the amount of CT and MRI pathology. The gold standard of diagnosis remains the histologic brain material obtained through biopsy or necropsy and the subsequent transmission to susceptible rodents. The brainstem and spinal cord are usually pathologically infected.

Recent data suggests the presence of prion proteins in immuno blocks of brain material is a sensitive specific marker for Creutzfeldt-Jakob disease. EEG is helpful in diagnosing this condition in dementia, though the EEG findings alone cannot determine whether one is having dementia or pseudodementia (associated wih depression).

B. WHAT IS THE PATHOLOGY OF THIS DISORDER?

ANS: A Proteinaeous infectious particle devoid of nuclide acid that is encoded by a single copy host PRNP, present in the short arm of chromosome 20. The function of the abnormal cellular PRNP gene is unknown, although both membrane forms exist, permitting transmittable neurodegenerative disease.

Experimental attempts to transmit Alzheimer's disease have failed, suggesting that an infective basis is unlikely. In some, a jerking contraction of various muscles (myoclonus) may occur in the presence of Alzheimer's disease, but this is unusual and should immediately raise the suspicion of Creutzfeldt-Jakob disease.

C. WHAT ARE THE DIFFERENTIAL DIAGNOSES OF MYOCLONUS?

ANS: It is lipid storage disease, encephalitis, metabolic encephalopathies due to respiratory failure, liver failure and electrolyte imbalance. Therapy for myoclonus include baclofen and valproic acid.

Q 121

A 29-year-old girl, an engineering student, has a habit of inducing vomiting after meals and takes diuretics in order to lose weight. For the last three years, she has been having problems with her concentration. Although her grade point average is high and she is in the top 1% of her class, she does not have adequate confidence to socialise freely. She is afraid of being fat and has undergone psychotherapy, but this does not appear to have helped. She admits to the psychologist that she cannot help herself when she induces vomiting. She has poor teeth and scratch marks on her knuckles. Two days ago, when she induced vomiting, she experienced diplopia.

On examination, she has impaired upward gaze and adduction of the left eye on the left lateral gaze.

A. WHAT IS THE DIAGNOSIS?

ANS: This patient has Wernicke's disease as a result of Bulimia.

Full-blown Beri-beri occurs rarely, although suggestions of disordered cardiovascular functions such as tachycardia, exertional dyspnoea, postural hypotension and minor electrocardiographic abnormalities are common. Occasionally, the patient dies suddenly, the mode of death suggesting cardiovascular collapse.

Ocular palsies may begin to improve within hours after the administration of thiamine and practically always within several days. Failure to respond in this manner raises doubts over the diagnosis of Wernicke's disease. Ptosis, 6th nerve palsy, and vertical gaze palsy recover completely within a week or two. Vertical gaze evoked nystagmus may persist for months. Horizontal gaze palsy recovers completely in nearly all patients, but a fine horizontal gaze evoked nystagmus often remains as permanent sequelae of the disease.

It must be emphasised that Wernicke's disease and Korsakoff phychosis are not separate diseases, but the changing ocular and ataxic signs and the transformation of the global confusional state into an amnestic syndrome which are successive stages in the recovery of a single disease process. In other words, Korsakoff's psychosis is the psychiatric component of Wernicke's disease. Wernicke's disease when the amnestic state is not evident is called the Wernicke-Korsakoff syndrome when both the ocular, ataxic symptoms are predominantly present.

In untreated cases of Wernicke's disease, there is elevation of the blood pyruvate and a marked reduction in the blood transketolase (a thiamine-dependent enzyme of the HMP shunt). One should not initiate treatment of a severely depleted alcoholic with an intravenous infusion of glucose solution. Such an infusion may exhaust the patient's reserve of vitamin B and precipitate Wernicke's disease in the previously unaffected patient or cause rapid worsening of an early form of the disease. For this reason, intramuscular or intravenous vitamin B should be administered to all alcoholic patients requiring parenteral glucose. The cardiovascular status of each patient should be monitored carefully. As these patients are confused and forgetful, they must be monitored continually.

The amnestic defect is related to lesion in the diancephalon, especially those of the dorsomedial nuclei of the thalamus.

A 36-year-old Taekwondo expert noticed his pupils were not equal in size. He is one of the contenders for the International Taekwondo (martial arts) competition. Yesterday afternoon he had felt a severe stabbing pain in his neck after a Taekwondo tournament.

On examination, he has multiple bruises from the fight and the left pupil is smaller than the right. There is ptosis on the left. Ocular movements are full in all directions of gaze and the rest of the cranial nerves are normal. Apart from an old healed fracture of his ribs from a fight six years ago, he has no organomegaly and the chest is clear on auscultation.

A. WHAT IS THE DIAGNOSIS?
ANS: This patient has a left Horner's syndrome, secondary to a left carotid artery dissection.

Minor, sometimes unnoticed, neck trauma can induce dissection (stripping of the intima or the media) of the internal carotid or the vertebral arteries: Chiropractic neck manipulation accounts for some cases. Severe blunt trauma, like a kick to the neck, can initiate a dissection several centimetres above the origin of the internal or the vertebral arteries.

The diagnosis may be confirmed by magnetic resonance angiography. In carotid dissection, transient monoocular blindness or TIA often precedes embolic or low flow watershed infarction, leaving time for therapeutic intervention. Surgical exploration is only considered for patients with increasingly severe TIAS or when a mild stroke is worsening. After the patient's symptoms are stabilised, anticoagulation with warfarin is recommended for six months. Repeat angiography often demonstrates a reestablished lumen in the formerly occluded vessel.

Q 123

A 35-year-old professional magician has just returned from a tour of Pakistan with a 3-day history of confusion, preceded by three weeks of generalised malaise, headache and vomiting. He found himself in the wrong train station and missed the train severals days ago. His wife has had to drive miles to pick him up and he appears confused and not his usual self.

On examination, he is febrile and irritable. There is a left-sided 12th nerve palsy.

- CT scan – Mild hydrocephalus
- CSF findings are as follows:
  - Opening pressure – 25 cm H_2O
  - Red cells – less than 1/mm^3
  - White cells – 160/mm^3 (7% mononuclear cells, 20% polymorphs)
  - Proteins – 2.5 g/L
  - Glucose – 1.2 mmol/L (blood glucose 3.6 mmol/L)
  - Gram stain – negative

A. WHAT IS THE MOST LIKELY DIAGNOSIS?

ANS: This patient has tuberculous meningitis.

The CSF should be subjected to the Ziehl-Neelsen stain for acid fast bacilli and culture. The patient should be started on rifampicin, isoniazid, pyrazinamide and ethhambutol. The possible complications are hydrocephalus, spinal block, recurrent seizures, deafness, hemiparesis and psychiatric disturbances.

A 13-year-old girl, suffering from gross acne vulgaris, complains of seeing double, photophobia and left periorbital oedema.

On examination, the left pupil is fixed and dilated with complete ophthalmoplegia of the left eye in all directions of gaze. Fundoscopy reveals papilloedema on the left and there is decreased sensation over the left upper face. She has fever and appears drowsy.

A. What is the diagnosis?
Ans: This patient has cavernous sinus thrombosis as a consequence of squeezing her spots. If this is not treated adequately, it will progress to exophthalmos, optic nerve compression and visual failure.

Cranial nerves III, IV, V and VI pass through the cavernous sinus. Weakness of the extra-ocular muscles, due to the involvement of cranial nerve III, IV and VI, is common. Since the VI nerve is the only cranial nerve traversing the inferior portion of the cavernous sinus, lateral gaze palsy may be an early neurological finding. Papilloedema, venous engorgement or a chance in mental status is observed in 55 – 65% of patients. Meningitis, often confusing the diagnostic issue, is present in 40% of cases, usually secondary to retrograde spread of thrombophlebitis. A quarter of patients will have dilated or sluggishly reacting pupils, decreased visual acuity (frequently progressing to blindness) and dysfunction of the V cranial nerve. With the spread of infection to the opposite cavernous sinus, these findings may be duplicated in the opposite eye.

Septic cavernous thrombosis may present itself in two ways. In the acute version, the onset between the primary infection (usually a facial cellulitis or squeezing of acne) and cavernous sinus thrombosis is less than one week. The patient appears seriously ill with a rapid worsening of symptoms and signs as described above and progresses to bilateral eye signs. On the other hand, some patients have a more indolent form of cavernous sinus thrombosis, usually secondary to dental infection, otitis media or paranasal sinusitis. The orbital manifestations are less impressive and involvement of the contralateral eye is late and an inconsistent finding.

Headache is the prominent finding (experienced by more than 80% of patients) with septic lateral sinus thrombosis, but acute nausea, vomiting and vertigo are often present since otitis media is a common predisposing condition.

B. WHAT ARE THE USUAL PREDISPOSING CONDITIONS FOR THE DEVELOPMENT OF THIS DISORDER?

ANS: Conditions predisposed to the development of cavernous sinus thrombosis are parasanal sinusitis (especially frontal, ethmoidal or sphenoidal) or infections as follows:

i) Staphylococci, aerobic or microaerophilic streptococci, gram negative bacilli, anaerobes with sinusitis.

ii) Staphylococcus aureus secondary to facial infection; otitis media or mastoiditis may be complicated by development of lateral sinus thrombosis or infection of the superior and inferior petrosal sinuses.

The most likely infecting microorganism depends on the associated primary conditions. Staphylococcus aureus is the most important associated pathogen in patients with cavernous sinus thrombosis and has been isolated in more than two-thirds of cases. This predominance reflects the importance of organisms in the associated infection of the face and scalp and in acute sphenoid sinusitis. Less commonly found in patients with cavernous sinus are streptococci, pneumococci, gram negative bacilli and bacteroides.

C. HOW WOULD YOU CONFIRM THE DIAGNOSIS?

ANS: MRI and CT scan are usually adequate, but suspicion of thrombophlebitis despite an equivocal report requires carotid enterography with venous phase studies. Enterography should show a narrowing of the intracavernous segment of the carotid sinus in the cavernous sinus thrombosis. Orbital phenography may also be useful and is the most definitive method of demonstrating cavernous sinus thrombosis.

In this focal suppurative intracranial process, the lumbar puncture will be diagnostic.

D. How should this patient be treated?

Ans: In cavernous sinus thrombosis, a potent antistaphylococcal agent such as nafcillin should be used, with vancomycin or linezolid reserved for the penicillin allergic patients and when methicillin-resistant organisms are suspected or proven. Combination regimens, including nafcillin or vancomycin plus metronidazole and a third generation cephalospbrin, are often required for optimal therapy. Surgical drainage of an infected sinus is necessary when antimicrobial therapy alone is ineffective.

Operative intervention of patients with cavernous sinus thrombosis is often employed, especially in a setting of sphenoid sinusitis. Internal jugular vein ligation and thrombectomy had been utilised in patients with lateral sinus thrombosis, but the efficacy of these procedures is poorly defined.

Anticoagulants are controversial as this is an infective process. Although anticoagulants prevent the spread of thrombus, the benefit is most apparent when initiated early during the course. The hazards of intracranial haemorrhage, including bleeding from the site of cortical venous infarction, must be recognised. In the absence of definitive data and specific contraindications, anticoagulation is most likely to be useful early in the course of cavernous sinus thrombosis. Anticoagulant is not recommended for septic lateral sinus thrombophlebitis because the cortical veins overlying the infected mastoid may become blocked, resulting in small venous haemorrhagic infarcts leading to an intracerebral haemorrhage.

E. What is the unique nature of this condition if the patient is diabetic?

Ans: Cavernous sinus thrombosis may occur as a consequence of mucormycosis causing cavernous sinus thrombosis when orbital invasion occurs. Without treatment, death may occur in a few days to a few weeks.

Mucormycosis originating in the nose and paranasal sinuses produce a characteristic clinical picture. Low-grade fever, dull sinus pain, sometimes nasal congestion or thin bloody nasal discharges, are followed in a few days by diplopia, fever and drowsiness. Examination reveals a unilateral generalised reduction of ocular motion, chemosis and proptosis. The nasal turbinates on the involved side may be dusky red or necrotic. A sharply delineated area of necrosis, strictly respecting the midline, may appear in the hard palate. With mucormycosis, the skin of the cheek may become inflamed. Fungal invasion of the globe or the opthalmic artery leads to blindness.

Opacification of one or more sinuses is found on CT scan or by MRI. A carotid arteriogram may show invasion or obstruction of the carotid siphon. Coma is due to direct invasion of the frontal lobe by mucormycosis. Early symptoms mimic sinusitis. Clouding of the sensorium may be attributed to diabetic acidosis. Rhinocerebral mucormycosis is a rare infection which usually develops in a patient during or following an episode of diabetic ketoacidosis. Onset is sudden with periorbital and perinasal swelling, pain, bloody nasal discharge and increased lacrimation. The nasal mucosa and underlying tissues become black and necrotic.

Intravenous amphotericin B is valuable in cranial fascial mucormycosis and should be employed in other forms of mucormycosis as well. Strict control of diabetes mellitus and decreasing the dose of immunosuppresive drugs, should they be on them, would aid in treatment. The drug is continued for up to 12 weeks. Appropriate management results in a cure of about 50% of such patients.

Q 125

A 33-year-old politician has noticed a blurring of his right eye and decreased libido over the last three months. Visual acuity and his perception of colour are maintained in both eyes, but there is a right upper outer quandrantanopia. The physical examination is, otherwise, normal.

A. WHAT IS THE DIAGNOSIS?

ANS: This patient has a prolactinoma which causes progressive visual failure and the optic chiasma is being compressed from below.

The size of the prolactinoma correlates with hormonal output. In general, the larger the tumour, the higher are the prolactin levels. Large pituitary tumours with a modest prolactin elevation are not true prolactinomas and differ in their biological behaviour.

The majority of patients with a prolactinoma have only minimal or no rise in prolactin in response to TRH compared to the normal rise of 200% or more, and the intermediate response (usually a doubling of serum prolactin) in patients with hypothalamic disease and those on dopamine blocking agents. The diagnosis may be made by a CT scan of the pituitary fossa or an MRI. Prolactin should be measured as there is a progressive visual failure and early drug treatment can be instituted should there be a prolactinoma.

Cranial pharyngioma should be considered in this age group, but it usually compresses the ciasma from above, producing a bitemporal field defect and beginning in the lower quandrants.

B. HOW SHOULD THIS PATIENT BE TREATED?
ANS: Transsphenoidal surgery of pituitary microdenoma is safe and frequently corrects the hormonal over secretion.

Hormonal over production is corrected in 24–75% of patients with Cushing's disease due to corticotrope microadenomas, and acromegaly, correcting the growth hormone concentration to less than 40 µgram/L.

Pituitary surgery is less successful with larger secretory tumours. In patients with serum prolactin concentration of more than 200 µg/L or growth hormone concentration of more than 40 µg/L, hormone concentration returns to normal only in 30% following surgery. Surgery is successful in up to 60% of patients with Cushing's disease due to corticotrope macroadenoma. The recurrent rate with this secretory macroadenoma after surgery induced remission is uncertain.

In the case of prolactin secreting tumours, hyperprolactinaemia recurs in 10–80% of patients. Although visual field abnormalities are usually reversible with surgery, cure of the tumour is unlikely. The intracellular portion of the tumour invading the cavernous sinus may be debulked, but parasellar extension remains. The early series noted an 85% symptomatic recurrence (due to structural interference such as visual defects) over 10 years in patients treated with surgery alone. When radiation therapy was used in combination with surgery, the 10-year recurrence was 15%. Bromocriptine (or other dopamine agonists) is the therapy of choice for macroprolactinomas.

Ten to fifteen percent of tumours shrink with bromocriptine therapy, but the numbers who stabilise without therapy is not known. Surgical removal of a prolactinoma is rarely curative, although surgical debulking may be indicated for a large tumour that causes mass effect. Prolactinomas in women and corticotrophoadenomas in both sexes are usually diagnosed while still microadenomas. In contrast, a majority of patients with acromegaly and most with prolactinomas have macroadenomas at the time of diagnosis.

It must be remembered that prolactinomas may grow during pregnancy and 15% of prolactinoma patients are first diagnosed in the postpartum period. Women with prolactinomas who desire pregnancy need special consideration. Medical therapy of patients with microprolactinoma results in uneventful pregnancy in up to 98% of the time. The remainder may develop hormonal or neurological disturbance due to tumour enlargement that rarely requires therapy.

Q 126

A 35-year-old newscaster for a satellite network is diagnosed with AIDS four years ago. She takes AZT, a protease inhibitor and nebulised pentamidine. She gets episodes of thrush which responds well with tropical antifungal agents, but has recently begun to notice pain in her hands, increased clumsiness with a propensity to drop things, and weakness on climbing the stairs.

Clinical examination do not reveal any abnormality, except some woolly spots on fundoscopy.

- Hb – 9.1 g/dl
- WBC – 2.8 x 10^9/L
- Platelets – 106 x 10^9/L
- MCV – 98.9 fl
- CPK – 654 IU/L

A. What are the diagnoses?
Ans: This patient has zidovidine induced bone marrow suppression, and proximal myopathy. Both conditions would be relieved by stopping the drug.

She may also have AIDS related neuropathy which is characteristically painful.

Q 127

A 42-year-old African political dissident was diagnosed as having AIDS three years ago.

He has been losing weight and is taking zidoyudine, a protease inhibitor, dapsone and pyrimethamine. He has had an episode of pheumocystis carinii which reponded well to therapy and he has been prophylaxis since. He has a 2-week history of dysphagia which did not respond to fluconazole.

- Hb – 9.3 g/dl
- WBC – 3.5 x 10/L,
- Neutrophils – 0.8 x 10⁹/L
- Platelets – 87 x 10⁹/L
- Endoscopy reveals a deep ulcer in the lower third of the oesophagus.

A. WHAT IS THE MOST LIKELY DIAGNOSIS?
ANS: This patient has CMV ulceration caused by bone marrow suppression.

The eyes should be examined for early changes of CMV retinitis. He should be treated with foscanet. Ganciclovir should not be used as it is myelosuppressive. Another advantage of using foscanet is it does not predispose to retinal detachment, unlike ganciclovir.

Q 128

A 60-year-old lady forensic pathologist is found to be HIV positive. Eight months later she experiences several weeks of fever and mild exertional breathlessness. She also complains of a sharp discomfort in the chest, aggravated on inspiration and worsened by lying down and leaning backwards.

On examination, she has a temperature of 37.7°C and tachycardia. The rest of the examination is normal, except for oral hairy leucoplacia and a film violet plaque over her left shin. Histology confirms this to be Kaposi's sarcoma.

- Hb – 10.4 g/dl
- WBC – 8.1 x 10⁹/L
- Platelets – 149 x 10⁹/L
- Sodium – 137 mmol/L
- Potassium – 3.6 mmol/L
- Urea – 3.3 mmol/L

- Creatinine – 37 μmol/L
- Bilirubin – 16 μmol/L
- ALT – 131 IU/L
- AST – 78 IU/L
- Albumin – 37 g/L
- Chest X-ray – A large heart with no abnormality of the lung-field.
- SaO_2 – 97% on air

A. What is the most likely diagnosis?
Ans: This patient has tuberculous pericarditis, which occurs early in the initial phase of HIV.

This is readily suggested by the ECG which shows a characteristic generalised ST elevation in almost all leads and a depression of the PQ interval. The ST elevation has a charactistic boat like morphology. Echocardiography will confirm it.

The appearance of fever and precordial pain at about the same time, often 1–2 weeks after a viral illness, is an important feature in the differentiation of acute pericarditis and myocardial infarction. The ST segment alterations on the ECG are usually transitory, but the abnormal T-waves may persist for several years or indefinitely and be a source of confusion in persons without a clear history of pericarditis. Pleuritis and pneumonitis frequently accompany pericarditis. Such patients should be advised to rest.

A common diagnostic error is assuming that the acute viral or idiopathic pericarditis represents acute myocardial infarction and vice versa. Acute pericarditis may complicate the viral, pyogenic, mycobacterial and fungal infections that occur with AIDS.

Q 129

A 31-year-old pilot for Air India has dry cough, fever and headache. She had been saddened to discover that her 7-month old daughter, who had an intractable lung infection, is infected with HIV.

On examination, she appears ill and has a temperature of 37.8°C. She is slightly drowsy, but orientated. There is neck stiffness, no photophobia and no neurological signs are detected. She has several mildly enlarged, non-tender lymph nodes in the neck and axillary region. The rest of the examination is unremarkable. She noticed some blurring of the vision, but a fundoscopy reveals nothing except some cotton wool spots.

- Hb – 9.7 g/dl
- WBC – 5.2 x 10⁹/L
- Platelets – 312 x 10⁹/L
- Sodium – 141 mmol/L
- Potassium – 3.9 mmol/L
- Urea – 5.6 mmol/L
- Blood glucose – 5.2 mmol/L
- Bilirubin – 17 μmol/L
- ALT – 153 IU/L
- AST – 71 IU/L
- Albumin – 35 g/l
- CRP – 48 mg/l
- Chest X-ray – Some diffused infiltration in the left mid-zone.
- CT scan of the brain – Normal.
- MRI shows multiple ring-enhancing lesions
- CSF-WBC – 57 cells/mm³,
- Lymphocytes – 85%
- RBC – 115 cells/mm³
- Protein – 0.5 g/L
- Glucose – 2.3 g/L
- No bacteria or fungi.
- SaO₂ on air – 94%
- Blood film tested for malaria parasites – Negative for three consecutive samples.

A. What is the diagnosis?

Ans: This patient has cryptococcal meningitis secondary to AIDS.

CNS infection is seen in up to 85% of AIDS patients with cryptococcal disease, a majority of patients showing signs of subacute meningoencephalitis. The MRI lesions are confirmatory. A high index of suspicion is essential in order to make an early diagnosis. Fever is absent in virtually all patients. Nausea and vomiting are present in about 40% and altered mental status, headache and meningeal signs are present in a quarter of patients. The incidence of seizures and focal neurological deficits is low.

Pulmonary disease is seen in 40% of patients, 90% of whom will also have CNS infection. A presumptive diagnosis of cryptococcal infection can be made upon identification of organisms in the CSF via an Indian

Ink examination, by measuring the presence of cryptococcal antigen in blood or spinal fluid, and by histological evidence of crytococcal infection in the biopsied specimens. A definitive diagnosis is made by culturing the organism from spinal fluid, blood, bone marrow, sputum or tissue.

Cryptococcal antigen is present in the CSF in virtually all cases of cryptococcal meningitis, although in 15% of cases all other findings may be normal. Therapy with amphotericin B should be initiated in any patient with evidence of crytococcal infection, either by antigen or culture. An alternative is flucytosine. Half the patients with flucytosine may have to be taken off the drug, at least for part of the course, due to neutropenia. With this therapy alone, half the patients will relapse. It is therefore recommended that at termination of amphotericin, patients be put on fluconazole 100–200 mg daily indefinitely. One should consider placing all patients with HIV infection on fluconazole 100–200 mg daily, as a prophylaxis against both candida and cryptococcal infection, once the CD4 T cell-count falls below 100 cells/microlitre.

Uncommon manifestations of crytococcal infection in patients with HIV infection include skin lesions resembling Molluscum contagiosum, lymphadenopathy, palatal and glossal ulcer, arthritis, gastroenritis, myocarditis and prostatitis (in males). Patients with CNS cryptococcal disease often display symptoms for weeks to months prior to diagnosis, as in the case with many AIDS associated opportunistic infection, a high index of suspicion is essential in order to make an early diagnosis.

Q 130

A 52-year-old Italian sales manager of a large toy shop, who injects heroin, is diagnosed on the basis of hairy leukoplacia and a positive ELISA to have AIDS. He has a 4-month history of increasing central and epigastric abdominal discomfort, nausea and vomiting.

He is afebrile and the examination of his abdomen reveals no abnormality. His customers have commented that the whites of his eyes appears yellow.

- Hb – 11.1 g/dl
- WBC – 4.3 x 10⁹/L
- Platelets – 253 x 10⁹/L

- Sodium – 139 mmol/L
- Potassium – 4.1 mmol/L
- Urea – 3.3 mmol/L
- Bilirubin – 46 μmol/L
- ALT – 671 IU/L
- AST – 69 IU/L
- Urine bilirubin – ++
- Urobilinogen – ++
- Abdominal ultrasound – Dilation of the common bile duct. There are no intraabdominal masses or lymphadenopathy.

A. WHAT IS THE MOST LIKELY DIAGNOSIS?

ANS: This patient has sclerosing cholangitis in association with HIV.

About one third of HIV patients show some biochemical evidence of biliary tract disease and CMV may cause a syndrome of papillary stenosis and sclerosing cholangitis. Kaposi's sarcoma lesions may infiltrate the gall bladder and biliary tree leading to a clinical picture of obstructive jaundice similar to those seen in sclerosing cholangitis.

Biliary tract disease, in the form of papillary stenosis or sclerosing cholangitis, has also been reported in the context of crytosporidiosis. Primary or idiopathic sclerosing is a disorder characterised by a progressive, inflammatory sclerosing and obliterative process affecting the extrahepatic and, often, the intrahepatic bile ducts. Therapy with cholestryramine may help control symptoms of pruritis, and antibiotics are useful when cholangitis complicates the clinical picture. Vitamin D and calcium supplementation may help prevent the loss of bone mass. Balloon dilation or surgical intervention may be helpful. Efforts of biliary-enteric anastomoses or stent placement may be complicated by recurrent and further progression of the stenotic process.

Primary sclerosing cholangitis is one of the most common indications for a liver transplantation. The mean follow-up time from the diagnosis of sclerosing cholangitis to transplantation is six years. In sclerosing cholangitis and Caroli's disease (multiple cystic dilation of the intrahepatic biliary tree), recurrent infection and sepsis associated with an inflammatory and fibrotic obstruction of the biliary tree may necessitate transplantation. ERCP or MRCP may be used to diagnose sclerosing cholangitis. Following retrograde cholangiography, the common bile duct should show a thickening of the wall with a narrow, beaded lumen typical of sclerosing cholangitis. Hepatobiliary ultrasound may be used to diagnose sclerosing cholangitis.

When obstruction cannot be relieved in sclerosing cholangitis, antibiotics may be helpful in controlling superimposed infection or, when administered on a chronic basis, as a prophylatic treatment in suppressing recurrent episodes of ascending cholangitis. Without relief of the obstruction, there is a steady progression to endstage cirrhosis and its terminal manifestations.

Q 131

A 34-year-old HIV-positive sitar musician is afflicted with a sense of fatigue. He was diagnosed as suffering from the chronic fatigue syndrome. He also complains of intermittent dizziness. There are no other complaints apart from an occasional sense of nausea.

He is afebrile, but appears clinically dehydrated with a postural drop of blood pressure ranging from 120/80 mmHg lying to 80/45 mmHg standing. The examination did not reveal any other abnormality.

Lab results:
- Hb – 10.3 g/dl
- WBC – 4.3 x 10⁹/L
- Platelets – 421 x 10⁹/L
- Sodium – 121 mmol/L
- Potassium – 5.8 mmol/L
- Urea – 7.9 mmol/L
- Creatinine – 118 µmol/L
- Glucose – 2.8 mmol/L
- Chest X-ray – Normal
- Blood culture – Negative
- Culture for mycobacterium avium intracellularae – Negative

A. WHAT IS THE DIAGNOSIS?
ANS: This patient has Addison's disease, most likely caused by CMV adrenalitis.

Postmortem studies show that 50% of HIV patients have CMV adrenalitis. A measurement of ACTH levels and testing of the adrenal reserves with the infusion of ACTH will provide a clear-cut differentiation when a diagnosis doubt exists. The patient should be rehydrated and the hypoglycaemia corrected. Hormonal replacement therapy should also be started. The hyponatreamia is due to loss of sodium into the urine, due to aldosterone deficiency, and movement into the cells. This extravascular sodium loss depletes extracellular fluid volume and accentuates hypotension.

Raised plasma vasopressin and angiotensin II levels contribute to hyponatraemia through impairment of water clearance. The hyperkalaemia is due to a combination of aldosterone deficiency, impaired glomerular filtration and acidosis. Mild to moderate hypercalcaemia occurs in up to 20% of patients. The anaemia of Addison's disease is masked by the plasma volume.

Q 132

An obese patient, diagnosed to have Picwickian syndrome, had his arterial blood gas examined.

The results:
- PO_2 – 9.2 kPa
- PCO_2 – 7.3 kPa
- pH – 7.35
- HCO_3 – 33 mmol/L

A. WHAT IS THE DIAGNOSIS?
ANS: This patient has compensated chronic respiratory acidosis due to the Picwickian syndrome.

In this condition, hypoxia stimulates increased ventilation. Carbon dioxide is more diffusable than oxygen. Excretion of carbon dioxide is enhanced, despite the barrier to gas exchange. This patient should not be given more than 24% oxygen during therapy as he is dependent on the hypoxic drive.

Q 133

A 36-year-old computer software engineer is admitted to Casualty with 3-hour history of severe right flank and loin pain. He has had red urine on several occasions in the last eight months. He is on no medication and is happily married with three children. His mother had died at the age of 53 from a stroke following a severe headache.

On examination, he appears pale, but afebrile. He has tender ballotable mass palpable in the left flank. His blood pressure is 192/122 mmHg. Fundoscopy reveals Grade 3 retinopathy and his heart sounds normal.

- WBC – 8.5 x 10⁹/L (with 62% neutrophils and 35% lymphocytes)
- Platelets – 326 x 10⁹/L
- Sodium – 137 mmol/L
- Potassium – 5.9 mmol/L
- Bicarbonate – 21.3 mmol/L
- Urea – 24 mmol/L
- Creatinine – 462 µmol/L
- Albumin – 35 g/L
- Calcium – 2.1 mmol/L
- Phosphate – 1.1 mmol/L
- AST – 23 IU/L
- Alkaline phosphate – 123 IU/L
- Urinalysis dip stick – Protein – ++
- Blood – +++
- Microscopy – red cells +++ no organisms, no cast.
- ECG – Voltage criteria for left ventricular hypertrophy by Sokolow's criteria.

A. WHAT IS THE PATIENT'S DIAGNOSIS?
ANS: This patient has adult polycystic kidney disease which is autosomal dominantly transmitted. This patient also has left ventricular hypertrophy secondary to hypertension, due to the renal disease.

Ultrasound and radioscopic renal scanning can reveal the cysts. This disorder is found in one in 500 autopsies and one in 3,000 hospital admission and it is responsible for 10% of endstage renal failure. The inheritance of this disease is linked in most families to the alpha-hemoglobin gene complex and the phosphoglycerate kinase genes on the short arm chromosome 16.

Hepatic cysts occur in one-third of patients. Cysts may also occur in the spleen, pancreas, lungs, ovaries, testes, epididymis, thyroid, uterus, broad ligament and bladder. It is probable this patient's mother died from subarachnoid haemorrhage from an intracranial aneurysm, which causes death or neurologic injury in one out of 10 patients, but routine cerebral arteriography is not necessary. Mitral valve prolapsed and mitral, aortic and tricuspid valve incompetence occur more often in control groups.

This patient is anaemic, but polycythaemia occurs occasionally in patients with solitary polycystic kidney disease, hydronephosis and artery stenosis.

Q 134

A 45-year-old schizophrenic who wanders from one veteran hospital to another, arrives in Casualty with lacerations on his face. He had been arrested for being a public nuisance and trying to snatch the purse from an old lady. The patient is disoriented and smells strongly of alcohol. No other abnormality is found on examination and the CT scan is normal. Six hours later, he is unconscious. His pupils are dilated, but react consensually to light. Oculo-cephalic reflex is present.

The fundoscopy is normal and there are no lateralising signs on neurological examination. His respiratory rate is 30/min, pulse 180/min and blood pressure 105/65 mmHg. There are bilateral basal crackles and heart sounds are normal. An abdominal examination does not reveal any abnormality.

Investigation:
- Hb – 16.7 g/d1
- Haematocrit – 0.56 l/L
- WBC – 10 x 10^9/L with 63% neutrophils and 31% lymphocytes
- Platelets – 416 x 10^9/L
- Sodium – 144 mmol/L
- Potassium – 6.1 mmol/L
- Urea – 11.2 mmol/L
- Creatine – 147 µmol/L
- Glucose – 8.5 mmol/L
- PO$_2$ – 12.8 kPa
- PCO$_2$ – 2.7 kPa
- HCO$_3$ – 6.1 mmol/L
- pH – 7.03

- ECG – Broad complex tachycardia
- Chest X-ray – Normal

A. WHAT IS THE DIAGNOSIS?

ANS: This patient has ethylene glycol induced lactic acidosis.

Ethylene glycol is an anti-freeze. It is a colourless, odourless, sweet tasting water soluble liquid used as a solvent for paint, in plastic and pharmaceutical products, the production of explosives, fire-extinguishers, foam, hydraulic fluids, windshield cleaner, radiator coolant and anti-freeze. Glycolic acid is responsible for decreased serum bicarbonate, metabolic acidosis and an increased anion gap, as well as for interstitial and tubular kidney damage. Glycolic acid contributes little to the toxicity of ethylene glycol.

The patient should undergo dialysis to remove the substance. Oxalate induced acute renal failure may occur as a complication of ethylene glycol toxicity. The diagnosis is suggested by the history of exposure to anti-freeze, in association with the coma, elevated plasma osmolarity and the large anion gap. Oxalic acid may precipitate as calcium crystals in the brain, heart, kidney, lung, pancreas, and urine, resulting in hypocalcaemia. The ethylene glycol and glycolic acid levels may be measured routinely. Oxalate crystals in the urine support the diagnosis. A faint, sweet, aromatic odour may be detected in the breath. Ethylene glycol is converted to glyoxylic and oxalic acid. In addition, this toxin creates metabolic blocks which may lead to an increase of endogenous organic acid. An increased osmolar gap, accompanied by back pain, hypocalcaemia and crystaluria, suggests ethylene glycol poisoning.

The patient should be treated with gastric lavage, activated charcoal and the airway should be protected. Seizure should be treated with phenytoin or benzodiazepines. Hypocalcaemia is treated with intravenous calcium salts and the metabolic acidosis should be corrected using sodium carbonate. Large doses are required. Fluids and diuretic may reverse oliguria, but does not enhance the elimination rate of ethylene glycol. Ethanol therapy may be necessary if there is an ethylene glycol concentration greater than 3 mmol/L, and acidosis, regardless of the absolute ethylene glycol concentration. Haemodialysis reduces the half-life of ethylene glycol from 17 hours to three hours and enhances the elimination of toxic metabolites thus improving survival. Thiamine and pyridoxine may also be beneficial.

Q 135

A 44-year-old West Indian polar bear expert, surveying the ecological system of the Arctic and monitoring the behavioral pattern of the bears, developed a sudden loss of vision in the left eye four years ago. He had a stroke which left him with a mild dysphasia. He has pain in the hips and he is on non-steroidal anti-inflammatory drugs. He walks around with a cane.

On examination, he is pale. His pulse is 90/min blood pressure 135/90 mmHg. Vitrous haemorrhage is noticed on fundoscopy of the left eye and proliferative retinopathy is visible on the right eye. Movement is restricted in both hips.

- Hb – 5.3 g/dl
- MCV – 110 fl
- WBC – 5.3 x 10^9/L
- Platelets – 236 x 10^9/L
- Sodium – 139 mmol/L
- Potassium – 5.2 mmol/L
- Bicarbonate – 18 mmol/L
- Urea – 36 mmol/L
- Creatinine – 610 µmol/L
- Urine dip test
  - Protein – ++++
  - Blood – ++
  - Microscopy – 120 red cells per power field, scanty granular cast.
- 24 hours collection:
  - Volume – 1,550 ml
  - Albumin – 3.4 g/1
  - Creatinine – 10 mmol/l

A. WHAT IS THE DIAGNOSIS?

ANS: This patient has sickle-cell disease and he requires treatment with folic acid as he has macrocytic anaemia.

The chronic therapy with the non-steroidal anti-inflammatory drugs has caused papilary necrosis and he has MPGN. The hypotonic and relatively hypoxic environment in the renal medulla, coupled with a slow blood flow in the vasa recta, favours sickling of the red blood cells which causes infarction predominantly at the apex of the medulla as this is the most hypoxic zone. This is worsened by non-steroidal anti-inflammatory drugs which increase the probability of the condition. MGPN is accompanied by proteinuria and nephrotic syndrome. The course of MPGN in patients is relentless, leading to end-stage renal disease. No treatment is effective. Transplantation is occasionally successful.

The diagnosis of the sickle-cell trait or any other sickle-cell syndrome depends on the demonstration of sickling under reduced oxygen tension. In the widely used sickle preparation, sickle-cells can be seen microscopically after the addition of an oxygen consuming reagent such as metabisulprite. Clinical means of achieving the same hypoxic condition is to tie a rubber band around the tip of the index finger and to take blood after a short period. The characteristic deformed red blood cell is diagnostic. Some laboratories prefer solubility tests which depend on the fact that deoxyhaemoglobin S has a low solubility, but a high ionic strength. These tests are reasonably specific for Hb S, although some of the unstable variants may give a false positive solubility test. Haemoglobin electrophoresis is performed to confirm the diagnosis.

The long standing pain in his hips is due to avascular necrosis of the femoral head. This patient should not be rehydrated. He should be given oxygen and folic acid. He should be warned not to take NSAIDs in future. Hydroxyurea may be given to raise the level of HbF and reduce haemolysis. Hydroxyurea increases the expression of the Hb F gene in patients with sickle-cell disease.

The long-term efficacy and possible detrimental effects of administrating agents that affect the expression of many genes are unknown. Hb F production may be stimulated by agents such as butyrate and recombinant erythropoietin. Malaria prophylaxis should be administered in endemic areas. The development of pneumococcal sepsis in children may be prevented by the administration of polyvalent vaccine and prophylatic penicillin.

Since patients with sickle-cell anaemia have an increased risk of developing infection, many of them trigger painful crisis, it is critical to detect it early and give appropriate antibiotics promptly. The blood of the patient should be taken for culture and sensitivity testing. The patient should be given a supply of opiates for analgesia. Some of these patients are at risks of becoming addicted to opiates.

Q 136

A 54-year-old archeologist is referred for deterioration in her hearing. She gives a 3-month history of malaise, a vague sense of weakness and episodes of aching girdle muscles. She is worried she might have caught something from the excavation site. These symptoms followed a non-specific fever which she was worried was malaria. She had started promptly on chloroquine. She always has a stuffy nose with occasional epistaxis. Subsequent films of malaria parasites were negative. Her hearing loss worsened the week prior to her admission and she had several falls which she attributed to her clumsiness.

On examination, she is pale, thin and has a temperature of 37.4°C. Both nasal orifices are encrusted and she has bilateral otitis media. On neurological testing, she has bilateral popliteal nerve palsy. She has purpuric lesions on her left shin.

- Hb – 9.4 g/dl
- MCV – 75 fl
- MCHC – 28 g/dl
- WBC – 14.7 x 10^9 /L, 77% neutrophils, 18% lymphocytes, 5% cosinophils
- Platelets – 534 x 10^9/L
- Sodium – 140 mmol/L
- Potassium – 5.3 mmol/L
- Urea – 19 mmol/L
- Creatinine – 48 µmol/L
- Alkaline phosphatase – 510 IU/L
- AST – 35 IU/L
- CPK – 160 IU/L (normal – less than 170 IU/L)
- CRP – 68 mg/ml
- ESR – 61 mm/h
- Anti-nuclear factor – positive in 1:38
- DNA – 23% binding (normal is less than 30%)
- C_3 – 83%
- C_4 – 77%
- CH – 90% (normal – more than 60%)
- Chest X-ray – A cavitating lesion in the right upper lobe
- Urine dip stick

- Protein – +++
- Blood – +++
- Microscopy shows dysmorphic red cells

A. WHAT IS THE DIAGNOSIS?

ANS: This patient has the Wegener's syndrome.

Pulmonary tissue offers the highest diagnostic yield for showing the presence of necrotising vasculitis. Renal biopsy confirms the presence of glomerulonephritis. The finding of elevated C-ANCAs supports the diagnosis.

Glucocorticoids alone offer symptomatic improvement with little effect on the natural history of the disease. The treatment of choice is cyclophosphamide. The leucocyte count should be monitored carefully during therapy and the dosage should be adjusted in order to maintain the count above 3,000/mm³, which generally maintains the neutrophil at approximately 1,500/microliter. With this approach, clinical remission can usually be achieved and maintained without causing severe leocopenia with its associated risks of cutaneous infection. Cyclophosphamide should be continued for one year following the induction of complete remission and tapered and discontinued there after.

The irreversible features of this disease are renal insufficiency, hearing loss, tracheal stenosis, saddle nose and impairment of nasal sinus function. Cyclophosphamide predisposes to cystitis in up to 43% of patients, bladder cancer in 4% and myelodysplasia in 2%. For patients who cannot tolerate cyclophosphamide, azathioprine is effective for some in maintaining remission. There is no firm data to support the use of trimethoprim sulfamethoxazole in Wegener's granulomatosis, although this is used in some centres. Methotrexate alternated with glucocorticoid has been shown to be effective in some patients with moderate disease.

Subglottic stenosis resulting from active disease or scarring occurs in 15% of patients. Ninety percent of patients with an active disease and up to 43% of patients in remission are positive for C-ANCA. Renal biopsies may miss the diagnosis since they frequently reveal segmental or diffuse necrotising glomerulonephritis, with or without crescents, in the absence of any extraglomerular vascular involvement. Relapse may be predicted by a rising titre or the re-appearance of autoantibodies.

Q 137

The two sets of results below were obtained six hours apart from a recently sacked 38-year-old police officer. He was filmed brutally hitting some demonstrators during a labour strike. His wife has faxed a letter stating that she wishes to divorce him and he is under a great deal of pressure from the bank to repay loans.

The first set of results:
- Sodium – 135 mmol/L
- Potassium – 3.1 mmol/L
- Bicarbonate – 20 mmol/L
- PO_2 – 12.3 kPa
- PCO_2 – 3.5 kPa
- pH (plasma) – 7.35
- Urinalysis – pH – 7.45

The second set of results:
- Sodium – 139 mmol/L
- Potassium – 5.5 mmol/L
- Bicarbonate – 13 mmol/L
- PO_2 – 12.7 kPa
- PCO_2 – 3.0 kPa
- pH (plasma) – 7.1
Urinalysis
  - · pH – 5.5
  - · Glucose – +++

A. WHAT IS THE DIAGNOSIS?
ANS: This patient has salicylate poisoning.

The specific assay for the plasma lactate is available if the diagnosis is uncertain. Plasma salicylate concentration in the toxic range (more than 2.9 mmol/L or more than 40 mg/d1) will confirm the suspected salicylate poisoning. Alkaline diuresis (an urine pH of 7.5 or greater and an urine output of 3–6 ml/kg body weight/hour) enhances the elimination of salicylates. Contra-indications for this mode of therapy include chronic heart failure, renal failure and cerebral oedema. Repeated oral dosing with activated charcoal (with sorbitol as needed to enhance gastrointestinal motility enhances the elimination of salicylates.

Salicylates slows gastric emptying and intestinal motility, have a slow dissolution and absorption characteristics. Salicylates create a metabolic block, which leads to the production of mixture of endogenous acids. Salicylates stimulate the respiratory centre directly, causing respiratory alkalosis as the earliest derangement in salicylate intoxication and may be the only acid-based dysfunction in some patients. Anion gap metabolic acidosis is characteristic of salicylate poisoning. This increased anion gap, metabolic acidosis, respiratory alkalosis, ketosis and tinnitus suggest salicylate poisoning. Pulmonary oedema (ARDS) may occur with salicylate poisoning. Radioopaque densities may be visible on abdominal X-rays following the ingestion of salicylates.

Common poisons whose effects are delayed in onset include cancer therapeutic agents, carbamazepine, carbon tetrachloride, colchicines, digoxin, disulfiram, ethylene glycol, heavy metals, lithium, methanol, monoamine oxidase inhibitors, mushrooms, some plants, narcotics, phenytoin, podophylline, salicylates and enteric-coated, slow or sustained release medications. Salicylates are effectively removed by haemodialysis, which should be considered with severe overdose, cerebral oedema, a failure of conventional therapy or a compromised renal or hepatic function. Salicylates are identified by a positive varied chloride test on either blood or urine. Salicylates uncouple oxidative phosphorylation and produce an increase in metabolic rate, oxygen consumption, glucose utilisation and heat production. They also inhibit the TCA cycle and block carbohydrate and lipid metabolism, resulting in metabolic acidosis and ketonaemia. Salicylates produce liver damage resulting in increased plasma activity and prolongation of prothrombin time.

Q 138

A 27-year-old gentleman, on a pilgrimage to visit the sacred shrines of Buddha, is admitted with a 4-day history of recurrent fever, muscular ache, headache and photophobia. He has been on anti-malaria prophylaxis, but has no other significant medical history except for an appendicetomy six years ago. Some of the sites, where he has to prostate himself, were flooded and he had walked through marshland.

On examination, he is febrile with a temperature 37.8°C. His conjunctiva are injected and the pupil demonstrates episceritis. His cervical nodes are enlarged and his splenic tip is palpable. He has neck stiffness, but no focal neurological deficits.

- The three malaria parasites screen – Negative
- Hb – 13.4 g/dl
- WBC – 15.1 x 10⁹/L, 91% neutrophils
- Platelets – 123 x 10⁹/L
- Sodium – 143 mmol/L
- Potassium – 4.2 mmol/L
- Urea – 16 mmol/L
- Creatinine – 185 µmol/L
- Bilirubin – 35 micromol/L
- Alkaline phosphatase – 548 IU/L
- AST – 47 IU/L
- Glucose – 4.7 mmol/L
- Urine dip test
  · Protein – ++
  · Blood – ++
  · Microscopy – Occasional granular casts
- CSF
  · Protein – 0.56 g/1
  · Glucose – 3.5 g/L
  · cells (neutrophils – 11/hpf; lymphocytes – 17/hpf)

A. WHAT IS THE DIAGNOSIS?

ANS: Leptospiral antigen may be demonstrated in the biopsies of the sites of muscle pain by fluorescent antibody.

In skeletal muscle, focal necrotic and necrobiotic changes typical of leptospirosis occur. Early in the course of the disease there may be swelling and vacuolation. Healing ensues with the formation of myofibrils with some minor degree of fibrosis. Glomerular lesions are either absent or comprise mesangial hyperplasia and focal foot process fusion which are interpreted as non-specific and is associated with acute inflammation and protein infiltration.

Microscopic alteration in the liver is not diagnostic and correlate with the degree of functional impairment. Special staining techniques using silver impregnation methods may demonstrate organisms in the luminal or renal tubules, but rarely in the other organs. Weil's disease may be due to serotypes other than leptospirosis icterohaemorrhagiae, and is defined as severe leptospirosis with jaundice usually accompanied by azotemia, haemorrhages, anaemia, altered consciousness and persistent fever.

The figures have been reported to be as high in a study from Portugal. This supports that the leptospira directly causes toxic damage to the target organ. Liver disturbances include tenderness in the right upper quadrant and a palpable liver, both of which are common when jaundice is present. The serum aspartate amino transferase (AST) usually does not increase beyond 5-fold, regardless of the degree of hyperbilirubinaemia in which the conjugated bilirubin predominates. It is interesting that among 201 patients in Singapore clinically suspected of having leptospirosis, 3% demonstrated serological evidence of hantavirus. Nephropathy is common in Europe.

It is recommended that blood be submitted for hantavirus serology in all cases of suspected leptospirosis.The patient may be treated with antimicrobials such as penicillin, tetracylcine, erythromycin or chloramphenicol. Human to human transfer is rare.

Q 139

A 32-year-old professor of astrophysics, also a body-builder, is admitted with abdominal pain. This started 18 hours ago and he is constipated. He has been on no medication, except an injection of anabolic steroids three years ago. He is normally active and can walk for miles.

Results:
- Full blood count – 14.3 g/dl
- WBC – 16.1 x 10^9/L (84% neutrophils)
- Platelets – 388 x 10^9/L
- Sodium – 137 mmol/L
- Potassium – 6.7 mmol/L
- Chloride – 101 mmol/L
- Urea – 7.8 mmol/L
- Creatinine – 113 μmol/L
- Glucose – 6.6 mmol/L
- Amylase – 785 u/L (normal – less than 180)

- Pa O_2 – 13.1 kPa
- Pa CO_2 – 2.7 kPa
- Anion gap – Increased

A. WHAT IS THE DIAGNOSIS?

ANS: This patient has a volvulus.

An X-ray of the abdomen may show dilation of individual loops of intestines which may be characteristic as in volvulus.

Erect and supine views will often show air fluid levels in the affected segments. Air under the diaphragm is best seen in the chest X-ray and is diagnostic of the perforated viscus, although it has also been reported in sports such as water-skiing. Air in the portal vein suggests intestinal necrosis secondary to mesenteric vascular occlusion. The diagnostic accuracy of the plain X-ray in all types of intestinal obstruction is about 75%. In patients with symptoms of incomplete intestinal obstruction, the physician can perform a small bowel enteroclysis by passing a tube into the proximal jejunum. The rapid installation of barium will distend the intestine and reveal subtle lesions missed by other tests.

The serum amylase is not elevated enough to make a diagnosis of acute pancreatitis. This patient requires an infusion of sodium bicarbonate immediately as this will bring down the potassium and correct the acidosis. The subsequent procedure to rectify this disease is laprotomy. The arterial blood gas shows a high anion gap which is compatible with severe acidosis.

Q 140

A 74-year-old man, in Nanking to research Japanese war atrocities, is admitted following an episode of haemetemesis.

On examination, he appears well, with warm peripheries, a pulse of 110/min and BP of 110/80 mm/Hg. He has tenderness in the epigastric region. Rectal examination confirms malaena. His only medical history is of hypertension (for which he takes beta-blockers) and he used to be addicted to cocaine.

Investigation:
- Hb – 10.3 g/dL
- WBC – 7.4 x10^9/L

- Platelets – 418 x 10⁹/L
- Sodium – 143 mmols/L
- Potassium – 4.9 mmols/L
- Urea – 10 mmols/L
- Creatinine – 154 µmols/L

He is treated with a H2-antagonist and gastroscopic examination reveals a gastric ulcer with a sentinel clot. This is promptly treated with a heater probe and a number of biopsies are taken around the edge of the crater.

Four days later the following results were obtained:
- Sodium – 143 mmol/L
- Potassium – 4.8 mmol/L
- Urea – 12 mmol/L
- Creatinine – 214 µmol/L

There is a disproportionate rise in creatinine compared to urea. Trimethoprim and cimetidine compete for excretion for the tubular secretion of creatinine and cause an increase in the serum creatinine, while sulphadiazine may crystallise in the kidney and result in an irreversible form of renal shut down.

A. WHAT OTHER CONDITIONS MAY CAUSE A SIMILAR BIOCHEMICAL PROFILE?
ANS: Other causes of an elevated creatinine, which is disproportionately high in comparison to urea, are liver disease, rhabdomyolysis, dialysis, pregnancy, vomiting and malignant hypertension.

Urea can diffuse back into the systemic circulation more easily than creatinine. Once it is filtered, the blood urea nitrogen rises more than serum creatinine. Normally, the ratio of the BUN to serum creatinine is 10:1.

Q 141

A 63-year-old train driver is referred six hours after the onset of severe back pain and weakness of the legs. He has a chronic cough, productive of clear sputum, and shortness of breath on exertion. He has had decreased urinary frequency and a poor stream for several years. He has not passed any urine since the onset of his symptoms. He has been treated for 16 years for hypertension and is currently on calcium channel blocker. He smoked 20 cigarettes a day during his teens and admits to 15 units of alcohol per week.

On examination, he is afebrile, his pulse is 115/min, in sinus rhythm, and the blood pressure in the right arm is 160/110 mmHg. The apex beat is displaced to the anterior axillary line and heart sounds are normal with a grade 2/6 pansystolic murmur. He has bilateral wheezes in the lung bases, his abdomen is soft with no bowel sounds, and a rectal examination indicates he has a smooth enlarged prostate. Bilateral lower limbs are pale and cold, with the femoral pulses impalpable. The tone is flaccid with no power, and reflexes are absent.

Investigation:
- Hb – 14.3 g/L
- MCV – 93 fl
- MCHC – 31 g/dl
- WBC – 5.7 x 10^9/L
- Platelets – 415 x 10^9/L
- Sodium – 143 mmol/L
- Potassium – 4.9 mmol/L
- Urea – 13.6 mmol/L
- Creatinine – 169 μmol/L
- CXR – Cardiothoracic ratio of 0.61; the lung fields are clear and there are osteophytes in the lumbar spine.
- ECG – compatible with left ventricular hypertrophy.
- Urine: (catheter specimen)
  - Volume – 70 ml
  - Proteins – trace
  - Inactive sediments

A. WHAT IS THE DIAGNOSIS?
ANS: This patient has a dissecting aortic aneurysm with anterior spinal artery occlusion.

Hemopericardium and cardiac tamponade may complicate a type A lesion with retrograde dissection. Acute aortic regurgitation may be found in over 50% of patients as a complication of proximal dissection. Transoesophageal echocardiography will readily diagnose the dissection of the ascending and descending aorta, but the blind spot of the TOE is the aortic arch.

Approximately one in 10 aortic aneurysms of syphilitic origin may involve the abdominal aorta, but these aneurysms tend to occur above the renal arteries, whereas arteriosclerotic abdominal aneurysms are usually found below the renal arteries.

Q 142

A 33-year-old lawyer is admitted for post traumatic stress disorder following an assault after she won a case sentencing a person for attempted murder. She had no premorbid psychological dysfunction and is on no medication. Her diagnosis of schizophrenia was made by the general practitioner and she was started on chlorpromazine. A week later she was discharged with an outpatient appointment for 3 weeks. However she was brought to the ward 3 days later by her partner from the law firm, who is concerned by her weakness and complaints of frequent headaches. The physical examination is normal and she was reassured. The next day the patient was admitted to casualty following a *grand mal* convulsion.

On examination, she is clearly in the post-ictal state with brisk reflexes but no lateralising signs and no meningism.

Investigation:
- Hb – 10.5 g/L
- WBC – 6.9 x 10^9/L
- Platelets – 344 x 10^9/L
- Sodium – 113 mmol/L
- Potassium – 3.5 mmol/L
- Urea – 3.7 mmol/L
- Creatinine – 69 μmol/L
- Calcium – 2.7 mmol/L
- Glucose – 4.5 mmol/L
- Urine osmolality – 91 mosm/l
- CSF:
  - Protein – 0.45 g/L
  - Glucose – 3.9 mmol/L
  - Cells – less than 2/mm^3
  - Lymphocytes per hpf – nil

A. WHAT IS THE DIAGNOSIS?

ANS: This patient has psychogenic polydypsia.

The rapid ingestion of huge quantities of fluid overloads the normal excretory capacity and produces symptomatic dilutional hyponatraemia, despite a normal renal diluting mechanism. Hyponatraemia of this type is diagnosed from the history of massive fluid intake. The patients are often women with psychiatric illness. Since water excretory capacity is normal, the urine is maximally dilute in this condition.

Hyponatraemia due to psychogenic polydypsia responds to water restriction. Rarely, patients with extreme hyponatraemia may require intravenous infusions of hypertonic saline. It is dangerous to replace sodium rapidly as this may cause central pontine myelinolysis. During deliberate polydypsia, extracellular fluid volume is normal or high and vasopressin is inhibited to a basal level because serum osmolality tends to be near to the lower limits of normal. Reabsorption of water from the convolute tubules and collecting ducts is reduced, so all the surplus water can be excreted into the urine.

Volume expansion raises the total delivery of sodium chloride in the water to the thick ascending limb of Henle and then to the medulla, all things being equal. It also raises renal blood flow and increases flow through the *vasa recta* reducing their ability to trap solutes in the medulla.

Q 143

A 27-year-old expert in zoology attends a clinic for contraception counselling. She records a BP of 190/100 mmHg and has had high readings during her last two visits. She has no medical history, except malarial complexes which had been adequately treated. She describes pain in her fingers and wrists during the recent winter, but took no medication. She has a progressive loss of scalp hair which is patchy.

She smokes occasionally and drinks social amounts. Her search for reptiles has taken her to many parts of the world. She has just returned from the Galapagos Islands and has undergone a series of immunisation.

She has a temperature of 37.5°C, and both wrists are warm and tender with a reduced range of passive movement. There are no dermatological lesions. Her pulses are normal and the rate is 80/min, regular and BP is 192/100 mmHg. She has a grade 2 hypertensive retinopathy. The apex beat is not displaced and she has a systolic murmur at the base of the heart, loudest on expiration. Examination of all other systems suggests normality.

Results:
- Hb – 8.3 g/L
- MCV – 110 fl
- WBC – 3.2 x 10⁹/L
- Platelets – 287 x 10⁹/L
- Sodium – 143 mmol/L
- Potassium – 5.5 mmol/L
- Bicarbonate – 23 mmol/L
- Urea – 27 mmol/L
- Creatinine – 318 μmol/L
- Albumin – 31 g/L
- Urine:
  · Blood – +++
  · Protein – +++
  · Microscopy – Red cell and white cell cast and numerous crenated red cells
  · 24-hour protein – 3.5 g
  · Radiology – Left kidney is 12.3 cm and right kidney is 11.9 cm
  · CXR – Normal
  · 2-D echo – normal
  · Blood cultures – Staph epidermidis in one out of three bottles
  · Urine cultures – No growth

A. WHAT IS DIAGNOSIS?
ANS: The patient has SLE with Coomb's test positive.

Although arteritis of large coronary arteries may result in myocardial ischaemia, there is also an increase in coronary artherosclerosis which may be related with hypertension of glucocorticoid therapy.

Libmann-Sach's wart-like lesions located at the angles of the A-V valves or on the ventricular surfaces of the mitral valves do not produce significant regurgitation.

Kidney involvement in SLE may range from 35% to more than 90% in different series. Sometimes it may lead to a fulminant inflammatory process leading to a rapid progressive renal failure. If immunoflourescence and electron microscopic studies of renal tissues are performed, abnormalities are found in almost all patients with SLE. Abnormal EEG occurs in about 70% of patients with SLE, usually showing diffuse slowing of focal abnormalities.

Glucocorticoids in low doses, salicylates or antimalarial agents are usually sufficient in patients with mild dysfunction. Non-steroidal anti-inflammatory agents may cause reduction of GFR and should be used with caution in patients with definite renal involvement. Serological data, including C_3 and C_4, should be followed serially. A return to a normal value of antibody to double stranded DNA or complements is encouraging and suggests improvement. The converse is not true; 85% or more can be expected to survive at least 10 years.

High dose short-term intravenous methylprednisolone reduces signs of systemic and renal activity and disease in patients with recent deterioration. Adjunctive use of cytotoxic agents, such as aziathioprine, cyclophosphamide or chlorambucil , exerts a steroid-sparing effect and may prevent progression of chronic lesions.

The positive anti-nuclear antibody test supports the diagnosis of SLE, but is not specific. A negative ANA test makes the diagnosis improbable, but not impossible. Antibodies to double stranded DNA (ds-DNA) and antibodies to SM are specific for SLE. The functional haemolytic component (CH-50) is the most sensitive measure of complement activation, but it is most vulnerable to error. Extremely low levels of CH-50, with normal levels of C_3, suggest inherited deficiency of a complement component, highly associated with SLE with ANA negative. It is interesting that this lady took antimalarial prophylaxis as this may reduce the severity of the haematological manifestations of SLE and lupus arteritis. Retinotoxicity is related to cumulative dosage, and ophthalmic examination should be performed annually should the patient be put on antimalarial drugs. The new biologics such as mycopheolate mofetil has radically altered the treatment of lupus nephritis and appears to significantly reduce steroid usage and may also be used in treatment resistant SLE.

B. How would her medical management alter should she become pregnant?

Ans: Pregnant women with SLE manifest of hypertension with proteinuria associated with a reduction in renal function and an absence of extra-renal manifestation.

The renal deterioration may be due to superimposed pre-eclampsia or the effects of hypertension or nephropathy, since there is no clinical evidence of lupus activity and no increase in entity and A antibodies. This is a critical distinction because these women may present with increasing hypertension when antihypertensive therapy or delivery, depending on gestational age and maternal condition is indicated instead.

Conversely, women with active SLE, who could be treated with glucocorticoids, are often delivered inappropriately early because of the mistaken diagnosis of pre-eclampsia. For the reasons described above, the management of patients with SLE during pregnancy should be coordinated with a rheumatologist.

C. WHAT ARE THE NEUROLOGICAL MANIFESTATIONS OF THIS DISORDER?

ANS: Any side of the brain can be involved in SLE, eg. meninges, cord, cranial and peripheral nerves. It may mimic multiple sclerosis. Mild cognitive dysfunction is the most common manifestation. Seizures may occur. Rare manifestations are psychosis, organic brain syndrome, headaches (including migraine), extrapyramidal disorder, lacunar infarcts, cerebellar dysfunction, hypothalamic with SIADH, pseudotumour cerebri, subarachnoid haemorrhage, meningitis, myelitis, optic neuritis, nerve palsies and sensory-motor neuropathy.

CSF demonstrates elevated protein levels in half of the patients and increased mononuclear cells in 30% of patients. Oligoclonal bands, increased Ig G synthesis and anti-neuronal antibodies may be found. CT scans and angiograms are likely to be positive when focal neurological deficits are present and less helpful in cases where there are diffuse manifestations. MRI is the most sensitive radiographic technique to detect changes of SLE; changes which are often non-specific.

Q 144

A 54-year-old translator for the United Nations, had been under dialysis for six years. Hemodialysis was changed after six years to peritoneal dialysis when he developed mild precordial discomfort, diagnosed as angina. Throughout this period, his only medication was tonics, Chinese herbal medicine and phosphate binders. In the last two years, he has been complaining of low back pain and hip pain when he has to sit for long hours to translate. His colleagues notice he has become irritable, has mood swings and appears confused at times. A radiology of the spine shows osteopenia and non-united fractures of the right suprapubic ramus and three ribs.

Investigation:
- Calcium – 2.3 mmol/L
- Albumin – 33 g/L
- Total protein – 61 g/L
- Phosphate – 1.78 mmol/L
- Alkaline phosphatase – 439 IU/L
- AST – 2.9 IU/L
- PTH – 0.85 mg/L (Normal – 0.73)
- Vitamin D – 63 pmols/L (Normal – 50–100)
- ESR – 36 mm/hour

A. WHAT IS THE DIAGNOSIS?
ANS: This patient has chronic renal failure with osteomalacia.

Bone biopsy will readily confirm the diagnosis of vitamin deficiency. Nitrogenous compounds of larger molecules are retained in chronic renal failure. It is possible these substances cause neuropathy, as patients treated with intermittent peritoneal dialysis have less neuropathy than patients maintained on chronic haemolysis despite the high levels of urea and creatinine in the blood of patients undergoing peritonal dialysis observed in some of the patients.

Correction of acidosis induced hyperkalemia with sodium bicarbonate is the treatment of choice. I.V. insulin and dextrose are useful in lowering serum potassium acutely, while iron exchange resins, calcium resonium or calcium polystyrene sulfonate, is useful in longer term control of hyperkalemia. The low calcium in CRF is due to the impaired ability of the kidney to synthesise 1.25 dihydroxy Vitamin D, the active metabolite of Vitamin D. This results in reduced calcium absorption from the gut. Serum phosphate begins to rise when GFR falls below 5% of normal. The low calcium elevates the PTH level, and the ability of PTH to mobilise calcium from bone may be altered. Despite hypocalcemia, tetany is rare unless patients are treated with excess alkali.

Renal and metabolite osteodystrophy are terms that encompass a number of metabolic, skeletal abnormalities, including osteomalacia, osteitis fibrosa cystica, osteosclerosis, and in children, impaired bone growth. Osteomalacia can occur, secondary to deposition of aluminium, in the calcification fronts. The sources are aluminium in dialysis and aluminium containing phosphate binding agents. In aluminiun induced osteomalacia, the serum PTH hormone is low and the calcium is often high. Chronic bone pain is severe and proximal myopathy often coexists, giving rise to gait abnormalities and impairment of ambulation. Arthropathy is associated with deposition of amyloid or beta 2 microglobulin. The cause of this is unknown, but may be related to elevated levels of cytokines in chronic dialysis patients.

This patient is also suffering from dialysis dementia. This is seen in patients who have been on dialysis for several years and is characterised by dyspraxia, myoclonus, dementia and eventually, seizures and death. Aluminium intoxication is probably a major contributor to this syndrome.

Q 145

An 18-year-old boy is brought in by his mother for weakness and laziness. His symptoms are attributed to the psychological effects of being bullied at college. He has complained of pain in the abdomen, which was diagnosed as worms and treated by a general practitioner. He appears as a normal, intelligent, articulate boy, but complains of polyuria. His BP is 100/52 mmHg. He is on no medication, but admits he has occasionally sniffed glue, but no longer.

Results:
- Sodium – 134 mmol/L
- Potassium – 2.3 mmol/L
- Creatinine – 43 μmol/L
- Bicarbonates – 36 mmol/L
- Calcium (corrected) – 2.37 mmol/L
- Glucose – 5.36 mmol/L
- Urinary chloride – 23 mmols/L

A. What is the diagnosis?
Ans: This patient has the Barter's syndrome, and magnesium and potassium should be replaced. The essential defect is reduced salt

(sodium chloride absorption by the thick ascending limb of the loop of Henle). It is characterised by high levels of renin, aldosteronone and bradykinin. There is resistance to the pressor effect of angiotensin, hypokalemic alkalosis and kidney potassium in the presence of a normal blood pressure. A role for prostaglandins has been suggested since PGE2 and PGI2 activate the release of renin and since the pressor response to infused angiotensin is blunted by the vasodilator effects of PGE2 and PGI2. The fluid depletion results in an increased delivery of sodium chloride and water to the distal nephron, causing an increase in renin which leads to an elevation of aldosterone, which in turn causes urinary Kallikrein activity, resulting in kalliuresis and hypokalaemia.

Hyperplasia of renal interstitial medullary cells (which synthesise PGE in culture) is seen. Indomethacin reverses virtually all the abnormalities, except hypokalaemia. Thus, prostaglandins, probable PGE2 and PGI2, may mediate some of the manifestations of Barter's syndrome. This syndrome may be seen as secondary hyperaldosteronism without any oedema or hypertension. The loss of sodium is thought to stimulate renin secretion and subsequent aldosterone production. There is a school of thought that believes an increased production of prostaglandins is not a primary abnormality since administration of inhibitors of prostaglandin synthesis only temporarily reverses the features of this syndrome. The weakness of perodic paralysis and polyuria is due to hypokalaemia. Hypomagnesaemia runs parallel with potassium and this is usually present. The inheritance of this condition is autosomal recessive and manifestations begin in childhood.

Barter's syndrome may be mimicked by magnesium deficiency, the over use of diuretics and vomiting. Magnesium depletion causes kalliuresis, diuretics cause potassium and volume loss, and vomiting causes kidney potassium loss and fluid depletion. The patient should be encouraged to increase his intake of salt and potassium. Potassium supplements may be required. Spironolactone, which antagonises aldosterone, can prevent potassium wasting, although salt intake must be increased. Inhibition of prostaglandin synthesis with indomethacin, ibuprofen or aspirin, has varying degrees of success. Beta-blockers may lower renin production.

It is interesting that magnesium production can cause potassium depletion due to increased renal and gut losses. Beta adrenergic catecholamines cause hyperkalaemia by stimulating potassium shift into cells. This phenomenon may be one of the factors leading to cardiac arrhythmias, causing death during stress or during treatment of asthma with beta adrenergic agonists. Reports of death of asthmatic patients associated with the use of beta-2 stimulants, cause great concern. However, salmeterol does not have this side effect as it has an exo-receptor site and intermittently stimulates the beta receptor like a telegraphic activation sequence in Morse code. Salmeterol has got intrinsic anti-inflammatory properties and does not cause down-regulation of the beta receptors.

Q 146

A 36-year-old newscaster has premenstrual discomfort. She is on the oral contraceptive pill and takes amphetamines at times when she needs to stay awake during her research . She has recently taken herbal medicine and trimethoprim prescribed by a doctor in mainland China as prophylaxis treatment for protection from an outbreak of chicken flu. She appears normal on examination and has been prescribed bendrofluazide for hypertension. Five weeks later she returns complaining of weight gain and pedal oedema.

On examination, her neck veins are elevated at 4 cm and she has bilateral pitting pedal oedema. Her pulse is 96/min, sinus rhythm and BP is 144/94 mmHg.

Investigation:
- Hb – 12.7 g/dl
- WBC – 12.1 x 10⁹/L (neutrophils – 63%, lymphocytes – 22%, eosinophil – 11%)
- Platelets – 313 x 10⁹/L
- Sodium – 142 mmol/L
- Potassium – 3.7 mmol/L
- Bicarbonate – 25 mmol/L
- Urea – 17 mmol/L
- Creatinine – 287 μmol/L
- ECG – Normal
- USG of abdomen – Normal size, unobstructed kidneys
- Urine:
  · Protein – +++

- Blood – +++
- 24-hour urinary protein – 3.5 g
- Microscopy – WBC casts and numerous RBCs
- Culture – No growth

A. WHAT IS THE MOST LIKELY DIAGNOSIS?
ANS: This patient has acute intestitial nephritis due to trimethoprim and thiazide diuretic. She should be treated with steroids.

The terms 'acute renal failure' and 'acute tubular necrosis' are zones of confusion. This is inappropriate as some are due to parenchymal disease, eg vasculitis, glomerulonephritis and interstitial nephritis can cause acute renal cell failure without tubular necrosis. The pathological term 'acute tubular necrosis' is often inaccurate, even in ischaemic or nephrotoxic renal failure, because tubular cell necrosis may not be present in up to 30% of cases. The trimethoprim and thiazide diuretic may cause acute renal failure by causing allergic interstitial nephritis. This interstitial nephritis is characterised by infiltration of the interstitial space by macrophages, lymphocytes, plasma cells, polymorphonuclear leucocytes and other cells, and interstitial oedema.

Common causes of allergic interstitial nephritis include antibiotics such as penicillin, cephalosporins, trimethoprim, sulphonamides, rifampicin, non-steroidal anti-inflammatory drugs, captopril and diuretics (thiazides). Acute renal failure may complicate interstitial nephritis, due to infections, neoplasia or infiltrative process. Pregnancy is suprisingly associated with an increased risk of renal failure, although the incidence has decreased with the improvement of obstetric care.

White cell cast and non-pigmented granular cast suggest interstitial nephritis and the broad renal granular cast of chronic renal disease is probably due to interstitial fibrosis.

Eosinophiluria (between 1–15%) or urine leucocytes is common in drug induced allergic interstitial nephritis. When studied using Hensel's stain (compared to Wright's stain), it is only 85% specific for interstitial nephritis. Similar eosinophiluria can occur in artheroembolisation, ischaemic and nephrotoxic renal failure, proliferative pyelonephritis, cystitis and prostatitis.

Marked proteinuria is found in approximately 80% of patients with allergic interstitial nephritis activated by cycle-oxygenase inhibitors. These patients have interstitial inflammation and a glomerular lesion almost identical to minimal change glomerulonephritis. A similar syndrome may occur with ampicillin, rifampicin and alpha interferon.

Predominantly non-glomerular diseases, such as acute hypersensitivity interstitial nephritis, may present features suggestive of acute nephritic syndrome.

Q 147

A 37-year-old woman, a game keeper in an African safari park, is admitted following a grand mal convulsion, which was preceded by 12 hours of confusion, irritability and poor concentration. Her work has deteriorated recently. Ten days prior to admission, coinciding with her periods, she developed a skin rash and headaches. She is on no medication.

On examination, she has purpura in centrifugal distribution. She is semi-conscious and the tone is increased. She has bilateral extensor responses. Examination of the fundi reveal bilateral haemorrhages. She appears pale. Her temperature is 37.9°C. No lymph nodes are detectable. Her pulse is 96/min in sinus rhythm and the blood pressure is 140/90 mmHg. Heart sounds are normal on auscultation and her chest is clear. An abdominal examination does not reveal any visceromegaly.

- Hb – 8.3 g/dl
- MCV – 100 fl
- WBC – 9.9 x 10^9/L, 63% neutrophils, 22% lymphocytes
- Platelets – 53 x 10^9/L
- Blood film shows schizocytes and crenated and helmet cells. Malaria parasites are not observed on the thick and thin smear from three consecutive samples.
- PTT – 13 sec
- KCCT – 43 sec
- FDP – Mildly elevated
- Fibrinogen – 2.9 g/L (normal 2–4 g/L)
- Sodium – 137 mmol/L
- Potassium – 4.1 mmol/L
- Urea – 14 mmol/L
- Creatinine – 196 µmol/L
- Albumin – 37 g/L
- Calcium – 2.45 mmol/L

- Bilirubin – 38 μmol/L
- AST – 35 IU/L
- LDH – 43.7 IU/L (mildly elevated)
- Glucose – 6.7 mmol/L
- CSF
  · 8 lymphocytes under gram stain
  · Protein – 0.46 g/L
  · Glucose – 3.6 mmol/L

A. WHAT IS THE DIAGNOSIS?
ANS: This patient has TTP and should be treated with fresh frozen plasma, aspirin and plasma exchange.

Haemolytic ureamic syndrome (HUS) and TTP (Thrombotic thrombocytopenic purpura). This is characterised by microangiopathic haemolytic anaemia and thrombocytopenia. The pathology affects the kidney and the central nervous system.

The combination of microangiopathic haemolytic anaemia, nucleated red blood cells, thrombocytopenia, fever, neurological disorders and kidney dysfunction, is virtually pathognomonic of TTP. The diagnosis is counter-intuitively supported by a normal coagulation test. TTP should be considered in all patients for whom the diagnosis is ITP or Evan's syndrome (ITP and haemolytic anaemia).

The involvement of the central nervous system is seen especially in TTP. The kidneys of patients with TTP exhibit a flea bitten appearance as a result of multiple haemorrhagic infarcts. Pathological changes are seen in the small renal arteries and afferent arterioles, which are almost blocked due to marked intimal hyperplasia, particularly in the TTP and fibrin deposits in the subintimal region. By immunofluorescent staining, complement components and immunoglobulins may be seen in the arterioles and fibirnogen deposits are present in arteries and glomurular capillary loops.

The intravascular coagulopathy seen in HUS and TTP may be a Schwartzman phenomenon caused by microorganisms or endotoxins, genetic predisposition and deficiency of platelet anti-aggregatory substances, eg. prostacyclin. Some patients improve after an exchange transfusion or plasmaphoresis, suggesting an accumulation of an unidentified toxin. Patients with HUS have more severe renal failure, often marked by oligoanuria and hypertension. In TTP, though the course may take months, kidney failure is usually less severe. The overall prognosis is poor in view of severe neurological involvement. In the management of TTP, high dose glucocorticoids and plasma exchange often provide complete remission and cure. Plasma exchange should be started as soon as possible and the treatment cycle can be repeated if thrombocytopenia recurs. Splenectomy and anti-platelet therapy have also been used with some degree of success in TTP patients. The success of plasma exchange in adults haemolytic uraemic syndrome is less well established than in TTP.

The LDH level is very high because of intravascular haemolysis. PT, PTT, fibrinogen concentration and the level of fibrin degradation product (FDP) are usually normal or only mildly abnormal. If the coagulation test indicates a major consumption of pro-coagulants, the diagnosis of TTP should be reconsidered. A positive anti-nuclear antibody is obtained in one out of five patients. The spleen and liver are usually not palpable. Neurological symptoms develop in 90% of patients whose disease results in death. These neurological symptoms may fluctuate and terminate in coma. The neurological findings may be focal seizures, hemiparesis, aphasia and visual field defect. Involvement of myocardial blood vessels may be a cause of sudden death in some patients. Although the exact cause of TTP is unknown, the mechanism is explained by localised platelet thrombi and fibrin deposition. Arterioles are filled with hyaline materials, presumably fibrin, and platelets and similar material may be seen beneath the endothelium of the otherwise uninvolved vessels.

Immunoflourescent studies have shown the presence of immunoglobulin and complements in arterioles. Microaneurysms of arterioles are often present. A high molecular weight form of Von Willerbrand's protein, as well as platelet aggregating protein, has been found in the plasma of patients with TTP. This may contribute significantly to the pathogenesis of the microvascular damage. Drugs used include glucocorticoids, anti-platelet drugs and some patients undergo a splenectomy.

The definitive therapy that produces an up to 80% complete response is plasmapharesis. The benefit of anti-platelet drugs (diperidamol, sulphinpyrazone, dextran and aspirin) is uncertain, but they are often used together with the therapy. Aspirin may increase the risk of bleeding and should be employed with caution. Vincristine may be effective in otherwise refractory patients. There is an ever present risk of sudden death, and therapy should be instituted properly. Even deep coma is not a contraindication to therapy since full neurologic recovery is the rule in patients responding to therapy. If treatment is instituted early, remission occurs in up to 2/3 of patients. Relapses have been noted in one in 10 patients, but this is usually responsive to therapeutic intervention. Platelet transfusions should not be given because they can precipitate thrombotic events.

Q 148

A 36-year-old restaurant owner has an increasing stutter. He has lost a great deal of weight during the last four months, but there is no complaint of any dyspepsia. Four days prior to admission, he had a progressive onset of left basal pleuritic chest pain, accompanied by a cough with green sputum, and in the last 12 hours he has been having dyspnoea. He has no history of any significant illness, except for hepatitis A. He drinks social amounts and smokes occasionally.

On examination, he is unconscious and his skin turgor is reduced. He has no cutaneous abnormalities and no lymph is palpable. The ECG does not show any ischaemic changes and the temperature is 38.3°C. He had a respiratory rate of 25/min and there are signs of consolidation in the left lung base. His pulse rate is 120/min and is regular; BP is 110/70 mmHg. Heart sounds are normal and an abdominal examination does not reveal any organomegaly and the neurological examination is normal.

- Sodium – 151 mmol/L
- Potassium – 6.1 mmol/L
- Bicarbonate – 7 mmol/L
- Urea – 24 mmol/L
- Creatinine – 147 µmol/L
- Osmolality – 379 mosm/l
- Hb – 15.4 g/dl
- WBC – 15.3 x 10^9/L (92% neutrophils)
- Platelets – 523 x 10^9/L
- PO$_2$ – 9.1 kPa
- PCO$_2$ – 3.1 kPa
- Microscope examination of the sputum – Gram positive diplococci
- CKMB – Normal
- Cardiac troponin – Normal

A. WHAT IS THE DIAGNOSIS?
ANS: This patient has diabetic ketoacidosis caused by the stress of infection with pneumococcal pneumonia. He has a type 1 respiratory failure and metabolic acidosis. This patient should be immediately rehydrated with antibiotics.

The blood glucose level will readily confirm the diagnosis. In diabetic ketoacidosis, due to hormonal abnormalities, acetoacetic and betahydroxybutaric acids, are produced more rapidly than can be metabolised. Severe ketoacidosis can occur in association with alcoholism. In diabetic ketoacidosis a variety of plasma acid base patterns may develop depending on the balance between production and renal excretion of ketoacid anions. There is an anion-gap acidosis in which the elevation in plasma unmeasured anion is about equal to the reduction in the plasma bicarbonate. DKA is often accompanied by abdominal pain and elevated total serum amylase levels, thus mimicking acute pancreatitis. The serum lipase and pancreatic iso-amylase are not elevated in DKA. Patients with DKA have elevated levels of PGE2 metabolites and diabetic animals have elevated levels of PGI2 which may play a role in the decreased vascular resistance and hypotension in DKA.

Rhinocerebral mucormycosis is a rare fungal infection which usually develops in patients following an episode of diabetic ketoacidosis. Organisms are from the general mucor, rhizopus and absidia. Onset is sudden with periorbital and perinasal swelling, bloody nasal discharge and an increased lacrimation. The nasal mucosa and underlying tissue become black and necrotic. Cranial nerve palsies are not uncommon. Proptosis, chemosis and retinal vein engorgement indicate carvernous thrombosis. Untreated, death usually occurs within a week to 10 days. Amphotericin B and aggressive debridement is the indicated therapy. DKA responds to insulin and most patients do not require treatment with alkali. However, when acidosis is extreme, IV bicarbonate therapy is justified. Hypertriglyceridaemia in a diabetic is associated with acute ketoacidosis. Such patients have hyperlipidaemia, elevation of VLDL, but not the chylomicrons. Occasionally, an elevation of triglycerides is seen with lipaema retinalis. In this case both VLDL and chylomicrons are present.

Q 149

A 25-year-old police officer has been passing reddish urine for the last three days. He had an attack of flu a week ago. This episode was associated with pain in the small joints of his hands which did not allow him to play the guitar. He has had a number of episodes of haematuria in the last two years. He did not report this as he takes marijuana and was afraid of dope testing. He has been losing weight and appears emaciated despite eating well and has had a protracted course of diarrhoea. He has no significant history and does not smoke. His wife is currently attending an infertility clinic.

On examination, he has pruritic vesicular rash over his buttocks and back which he has had on and off for a couple of years. There is no evidence of joint inflammation and his BP is 120/80 mmHg.

- Hb – 10.3 g/d1
- MCV – 76 fl
- MCHC – 7 g/dl
- WBC – 8.4 x 10^9/L
- Platelets – 323 x 10^9/L
- PTT – 20 secs
- KCCT – 35 secs
- Sodium – 135 mmol/L
- Potassium – 4.4 mmol/L
- Bicarbonate – 24 mmol/L
- Urea – 1 mmol/L
- Creatinine – 136 mmol/L
- Calcium (corrected) – 2.2 mmol/L
- Alkaline phosphatase – 3.3 IU/L
- Glucose – 4.6 mmol/L
- USG – Normal sized unobstructed kidneys; empty bladder
- Urine:
  - Protein – +++
  - Blood – Trace
  - Microscopy – Red cells and occasional granular cast
  - Culture – No organisms

A WHAT IS THE PATIENT'S DIAGNOSIS?

ANS: This patient has coeliac disease caused by malabsorption (iron deficiency anaemia and osteomalacia) and Ig A nephropathy.

A biopsy of the small intestine is valuable in the diagnosis of coeliac disease. It may show the less common infiltration of mucosa by amyloid and bacterial mucoproteins such as in Whipple's disease.

The infertility in this particular case is most likely due to the patient, as men with coeliac disease have a hormonal pattern typical of androgen resistance, characterised by elevated testosterone and LH levels.

Leakage of protein into the intestinal lumen may cause hypoproteinaemia and may be demonstrated by intravenously administered markers such as albumin labelled with iodine or chromium isotopes. A simple screening test for excessive fat in stools associated with malabsorption can be accomplished by the examination of the stool specimen stained with Sudan. The D-xylose absorption test is highly accurate in separating mucosal disease from pancreatic insufficiency.

Coeliac disease in children and coeliac sprue in adults are probably one and the same disorder with the same pathogenesis. It is difficult to estimate the incidence of coeliac sprue in any population because the severity of the disease varies greatly and individuals may have typical mucosal changes and have no overt or atypical symptoms such as in the patients described. Seventy percent of patients are women. The mucosa is damaged in patients with coeliac sprue and there may be a decreased release of pancreatic hormones such as secretin and cholecystokinin (CCK). This results in reduced stimulation of the pancreas with lower than normal intraluminal levels of pancreatic enzymes in response to a meal. In addition, the gall bladder appears to be resistant to the action of CCK, resulting in absent or minimal contraction of the gall bladder, which in turn leads to the sequestration of bile salts in an inert gall bladder. These two defects may result in an impaired intraluminal digestion of fat and protein. Dermatitis herpetiformis is an intensely pruritic, chronic vesicular disease characterised by symmetrical lesions distributed over the extensor surfaces, buttocks and back. Patients sometimes report that the pruritis has a distinctive burning or stinging component. The onset of such localised lesions reliably heralds the development of distinct clinical lesions 12–24 hours later.

Almost all dermatitis herpetiformis patients have subclinical gluten sensitive enteropathy and more than 90% express the HLA-B8/DRw3 and HLA-DQw2 haplotypes. Biopsy of the skin lesion will demonstrate immunofluorescence microscopic features of granular deposits of IgA (with or without complement components) in the papillary dermis and along the epidermal basement membrane zone. IgA deposits in the skin are unaffected by the control of the disease with medication; however this rash may diminish in intensity and disappear in patients maintained on a long-term gluten-free diet.

The discordance for coeliac sprue among HLA identical siblings and some identical twins raises the question of whether the additional susceptible gene (or genes) not yet identified, is required for the trigger of this disease. IgA nephropathy was described by Berger and Hinglais in 1968 as characterised by recurrent and gross microscopic haematuria. The diagnosis depends on the finding of prominent IgA deposits in the mesangium by fluorescence microscope. Berger's disease is the most common cause of recurrent haematuria of glomerular origin. It commonly affects older children, young adults, mostly males. A typical episode of macroscopic haematuria is associated with a minor flu-like illness on vigourous exercise. It is postulated by some that Berger's disease may be a monosymptomatic form of Henoch-Schonlein purpura.

IgA nephropathy recurs in transplanted kidneys in up to 40%. Such recurrences seldom result in a loss of renal function, but may be associated with haematuria. Patients with granular deposition of IgA in their glomerular basement membranes do not have circulating IgA antibodies and should be distinguished from individuals with linear IgA deposit at this site. The mainstay of the treatment of dermatitis herpetiformis is dapsone. Patients respond rapidly in 1–2 days, but careful pretreatment evaluation and close follow-up ensure complications are avoided. Dapsone may cause haemolysis and methaemoglobinaemia, but these are acceptable pharmacological effects of dapsone; a very low maintenance dose must be used to control symptoms and lesions. Gluten restriction can control dermatitis herpetiformis and lessen dapsone requirement, but this diet must be rigidly adhered to, to be of any benefit.

B. How should one manage the patient with coeliacs disease if he does not improve with the recommended dietary therapy?
Ans: If a patient with coeliac disease does not respond to a gluten-

free diet, other possibilities must be considered such as an incorrect diagnosis, noncompliance with the diet, another concurrent disease such as pancreatic insufficiency, ulcerations of the jejunum or ileum, lactase deficiency, collagenase sprue or, sadly, the patient may have developed intestinal lymphoma, a disease which appears more frequently in patients with sprue than in the general population.

It should also be considered that the patient may have developed lymphocytic or microscopic colitis. It must be emphasised that a small number of patients show a delayed response to a gluten-free diet, with significant improvements occuring only after 24–36 months of therapy. Approximately 50% of patients with refractory sprue respond to glucocorticoids. Such patients may also require parental hyperalimentation.

C. WHAT ARE THE ASSOCIATIONS OF THE PRIMARY DISEASE ASSOCIATED WITH THE CUTANEOUS DISORDER?
ANS: Coeliac disease is associated with dermatitis herpetiformis, diabetes mellitus, selective IgA deficiency, primary sclerosing cholangitis, primary biliary cirrhosis, ulcerative colitis and lymphocytic microscopic colitis.

Q 150

A 26-year-old aeronautical engineer has been admitted complaining of a sense of malaise and back pain for the last six months. He has had problems concentrating on his work as he complains of clumsiness, difficulty in swallowing and frequently gets into arguments with his colleagues. His wife, a psychologist, says he has changed. He appears to have manic depressive psychosis and exhibits bizarre behaviour.

Investigation:
- Sodium – 135 mmol/L
- Potassium – 3.1 mmol/L
- Urea – 2.1 mmol/L
- Creatinine – 83 μmol/L
- Chloride – 115 mmol/L
- Calcium – 2.1 mmol/L
- Phosphate – 0.8 mmol/L
- Albumin – 37 g/L

- Bicarbonate – 17 mmol/L
- AST – 87 IU/L
- Alkaline phosphate – 395 IU/L
- Urine dip test – No blood or protein is detected
- pH – 5.4

A. WHAT IS THE DIAGNOSIS?

ANS: This patient has proximal tubular acidosis secondary to Wilson's disease.

The neuropsychiatric disorder of this patient is due to copper deposition in the brain. The diagnosis can be readily confirmed by liver biopsy and he should be treated with penicillamine. Wilson's disease is characterised by cirrhosis, a softening and degeneration of the basal ganglia and pigmentation and the liver-cells are ballooned and show glycogen vacuolisation in the nucleoli. The liver shows all grades of change from minimal to severe periportal macronodular cirrhosis.

Wilson's disease is an autosomal recessive abnormality of liver excretion of copper, resulting in toxic accumulation of the metal in the liver, brain and other organs. Deficiency of the plasma copper protein, caeruloplasmin, is a characteristic feature. Sufficient copper may be released from necrotising hepatocytes to cause haemolytic anaemia. The syndrome is indistinguishable from schizophrenia, manic depressive psychosis and classic neurosis may occur as a result of metal deposition in the brain. Improvement in the psychiatric state can occur with pharmacological reduction of the copper excess; additional therapy may be required.

The locus of Wilson's disease is the long arm of chromosome 13 within 13q14-q21, and the close linkage between this locus and other map markers on this chromosome makes it possible to identify the carrier state and to make prenatal diagnosis in some families. The metabolic defect in Wilson's disease is an inability to maintain a near zero balance of copper. Excess copper, which is essential to life, accumulates because the liver lysosomes lack a normal mechanism to excrete into the bowel the copper which has been catabolically cleaved from the caeruloplasmin. This may cause a deficiency of caeruloplasmin, since copper excess in vitro inhibits the formation of caeruloplasmin from apocaeruloplasmin and copper. The capacity of hepatocytes to store copper is eventually exceeded, and a release into blood and uptake in extra-hepatic sites occur.

In Wilson's disease, more copper is present than can be bound by specific copper proteins. Such copper is as toxic as non-protein bound iron, zinc, mercury or lead. Death can occur from central nervous defects. In the brain, the excess copper is distributed ubiquitously. Necrosis of neurones with cavitations may be preceded with Opalski and Alzheimer type II cells. However, neither is specific for Wilson's disease. Increased copper in the kidney produces little, if any, structural change and usually does not alter renal function. Haematuria, proteinuria, Fanconi syndrome and proximal tubular acidosis (as in this case) can occur.

The Kayser-Fleischer ring in Wilson's disease are gloden brown pigments at the periphery of the cornea and characteristically broader superiorly and inferiorly than it is medially and laterally.

Type II (Proximal tubular acidosis) is a disorder where the bicarbonate reabsorption in the proximal tubule is defective and bicarbonate wasting occurs with a normal concentration of plasma bicarbonate. As plasma bicarbonate falls, the filtered load drops to a level where the defective tubules can reabsorb. Then the urine is free of bicarbonate and has a low pH. Potassium wasting and hypokalaemia occur, especially when elementary alkali is given, because bicarbonate is excreted in the urine, partly as potassium salt. Hypercalcuria is moderate and stone formation is rare. During the ammonium chloride NH_4Cl loading test, urine pH falls below 5.5. When acidosis is severe, bicarbonate should be given in large amounts, often more than 4 mmol/Kg of body weight and even up to 10 mmol/Kg/day because bicarbonate is rapidly lost in the urine.

Another approach is to use a thiazide diuretic and low salt diet, which induces milder volume depletion and enhances proximal bicarbonate reabsoption, thereby reducing the required dose. Potassium supplements are needed during therapy because excessive sodium bicarbonate reaches the distal nephron where much of the sodium is exchanged for potassium, which is then lost in the urine.

Q 151

A 50-year-old man is recuperating following an operation to remove part of the lungs for bronchogenic carcinoma. His postoperative recovery is complicated by severe legionella infection and he is admitted into the ICU.

- Urea – 24 mmol/L
- Creatinine – 925 µmol/L
- Potassium – 6.9 mmol/L
- Calcium – 1.73 mmol/L
- Phosphate – 2.3 mmol/L
- Albumin – 37 g/L
- AST – 965 IU/L
- Uric acid – 0.74 mmol/L
- Urinalysis dip test
  · Blood ++++
  · Microscopy – debris ++, no cells or casts.

A. WHAT IS THE DIAGNOSIS?

ANS: This patient has rhabdomyolysis causing renal impairment, and he should be treated by alkalinisation of the urine.

The dip test for blood could be positive either for haemoglobin or myoglobin. The mechanisim by which rhabdomyolysis and haemolysis impair GFR is unclear, since neither haemoglobin nor myoglobin is nephrotoxic when injected into laboratory animals.

Acute rhabdomyolysis predictably occurs with clostridial and streptococcal myositis, but can be also be associated with influenza, echo virus, coxsackie virus, Epstein-Barr virus and legionella infection. In fact, myositis, rhabdomyolysis and myoglobinuria have also been reported as complications of influenza infection. Although myalgia is exceedingly common in influenza, true myositis is rare.

Myoglobin and haemoglobin or other compounds released from muscles or red blood cells may cause acute renal failure via direct toxic effect on tubular epithelial cells or by inducing intratubular cast formation. Hyperkalaemia is common. This is particularly severe in patients with rhabdomyolysis, haemolysis and the tumour lysis syndrome. Hypocalcaemia can be symptomatic in patients with rhabdomyolysis, acute pancreatitis or following treatment of acidosis with bicarbonate. Haemolysis and rhabdomyolysis can usually be differentiated by an inspection of plasma. The latter is pink in haemolysis, but usually not in rhabdomyolysis, since free haemoglobin is a larger molecule than myoglobin, is protein-bound and filtered slowly by the kidney.

Legionella should be treated by azithromycin and rifampicin. Postoperative legionella is rare and it is possible that the air-conditioning system of the operating theatre or wards should be inspected.

B. What are the other causes of rhabdomyolysis?

Ans: Acute muscle destruction, rhabdomyolysis associated with myoglobinuria, occurs with acute toxic, metabolic, inflammatory infection and traumatic muscle damage. The molecular weight of myoglobin is lower than that of haemoglobin, so the urine, rather than the serum, changes colour in extensive rhabdomyolysis. Myoglobinuria causes a positive urine test for blood in the absence of urinary erythrocytes. A confirmatory test for myoglobin uses a specific immunoassay. Lovastatin alone, or in combination with gemfibrozil, has caused rhabdomyolysis and myoglobinuria. Alcohol causes acute muscle weakness with rhabdomyolysis and myoglobinuria by several mechanisms, including prolonged obtundation, seizures, hypokalaemia and hypophosphataemia. Chronic myopathy causing slowly progressing weaknesses is controversial.

Rhabdomyolysis should be suspected in a recent history of seizures, excessive alcohol or drug abuse, or muscle tenderness or limb ischaemia on physical examination.

Q 152

A 26-year-old woman has successfully undergone kidney transplant in China. Her regular treatment is cyclosporin A, azathioprine, prednisolone, frusemide and oral nystatin. She gives a 3-month history, after the transplantation, of an acutely swollen, hot, tender right knee joint. Examination of the aspirated fluid shows uric acid crystal and no organisms. She is prescribed regular allopurinol and a weekly course of indomethacin. A month later, she is admitted as an emergency case with a 16-hour history of fever, rigors and dyspnoea.

On examination, she has a temperature of 38.5°C. Her pulse is 130/min and blood pressure is 90/50 mmHg. Her JVP is not visible. There are signs of consolidation in both lungs. The abdominal and central nervous system examinations are normal. Her graft zone is non-tender.

- Sodium – 143 mmol/L
- Potassium – 4.9 mmol/L
- Bicarbonate – 25 mmol/L
- Urea – 11 mmol/L
- Creatinine – 141 µmol/L

- Hb – 10.3 g/dl
- WBC – 0.7 x 10^9/L (75% neutrophils and 25% lymphocytes)
- Platelets – 203 x 10^9/L
- Chest X ray – Bilateral parenchymal infiltrates
- PO_2 – 8.5 kPa
- PCO_2 – 3.1 kPa
- Urine microscopy – No sediments and no organisms

A. WHAT IS THE DIAGNOSIS?
ANS: This patient has allopurinol induced myelosuppression, causing pneumonia. The patient is also prone to other opportunistic infections and should undergo blood culture, urine culture, sputum culture, bronchoscopy with brocheoalveolar lavage and bone marrow aspiration.

   She should be treated with antibiotics and bone marrow stimulants such as growth colony stimulating factors (GCSF).

Q 153

A 67-year-old man, who teaches chemistry, has undergone a transurethral prostatic resection. Bladder irrigation was stopped after 20 hours, but was restarted again for a further 50 hours in view of the clot retention and the obstruction of the catheter. Recovery is uneventful.

Results obtained on the 4th day after the operation:
- Sodium – 121 mmol/L
- Potassium – 4.7 mmol/L
- Bicarbonate – 17 mmol/L
- Urea – 4 mmol/L
- Creatinine – 91 μmol/L
- Haemoglobin – 11.1 g/dl

A WHAT IS THE DIAGNOSIS?
ANS: This patient has hyponatraemic acidosis due to glycine.

Q 154

A 45-year-old French teacher is admitted for investigation of proteinuria and a deterioration of her kidney function. She has been paraplegic for 13 years following a fall off a horse. She takes baclofen and lactulose and practices intermittent self-catheterisation. She complains of pain, worse at night, in the forearm, aggravated by the wheel chair, and relieved by shaking her hands.

On examination, the skin overlying her right ischial tuberosity is chronically ulcerated. She has pitting oedema, her pulse rate is 80/min and the blood pressure is 130/90 mmHg. The heart sounds are normal. The peripheral pulses are all normal. She has a 6 cm, smooth, non-tender liver. She has spastic paraplegia with a sensory level at T11. Neurological examination is normal and her upper limbs are normal.

Results:
- Sodium – 137 mmol/L
- Potassium – 4.3 mmol/L
- Urea – 16 mmol/L
- Creatinine – 27 μmol/L
- Albumin – 28 g/l
- AST – 30 IU/L
- Alkaline phosphatase – 210 IU/L
- Hb – 9.7 g/dl
- WBC – 6.9 x 10^9/L (73% neutrophils)
- Platelets – 278 x 10^9/L
- Urine dip-stick – Protein – +++ 6 g/24 hours
- Blood – Trace
- Microscopy – Occasional granular and white cell casts, red cells and numerous white cells. Culture – Heavy growth of proteus
- Chest X-ray – Normal
- Ultrasound – Left kidney – 12.3 cm
- Right kidney – 12 cm

A. WHAT IS THE DIAGNOSIS?

ANS: This patient has amyloidosis due to chronic urinary tract infection. The diagnosis is readily confirmed on renal biopsy. Renal amyloidosis is a progressive disease for which there is no established treatment.

Remission may occur in secondary amyloidosis if the cause can be eliminated. Remission in primary amyloidosis is exceedingly rare; a few reports describe remission with the use of a combination of melphalan and glucocorticoids. Colchicine is of value in the prevention of amyloidosis in Familial Mediterranean Fever. The 5-year survival rate for patients with primary amyloidosis is less than 20%. Ezotemia, presistent nephrotic syndrome and myocardial involvement confer an even ominous prognosis.

Instances of amyloidosis have been reported accompanying infection, such as osteomyelitis, in which partial remission has occurred following treatment of the primary disease. There has been similar experience following successful treatment of tuberculosis or drainage of empyema. Many such reports are not substantiated by biopsy proof of resorption.

Q 155

A 73-year-old farmer is admitted at the request of his neighbour. He lives in a flat for the elderly and is normally independent. Over the previous five days, he had become progressively socially isolated, confused, anorexic and incoherent. The neighbours notice that he is often drowsy and he has been incontinent with urine on several occasions. He is on regular therapy for hypertension and has no significant medical history, except for gonorrhoea when he was in his mid-twenties. This was treated appropriately with no sequelae.

On examination, the man is unable to follow instructions. His temperature (axillary) is 38.2°C. Skin turgor is reduced. Pulse is 108/min, regular and blood pressure is 90/50 mmHg (lying). There is no abnormality in the major systems, in particular, no lateral neurological signs.

Results:
- Sodium – 160 mmol/L
- Potassium – 5.3 mmol/L
- Bicarbonate – 21 mmol/L
- Urea – 30 mmol/L
- Creatinine – 138 µmollL
- Plasma glucose – 10 mmol/L
- Hb – 16 g/dl

- WBC – 2.9 x 10^9/L (80% neutrophils)
- Platelets – 438 x 10^9/L
- Chest X ray – No abnormalities
- ECG – Lateral T-wave flattening
- Urinalysis – Protein – +++
- Trace blood

A. WHAT IS THE DIAGNOSIS?

ANS: This patient has urinary tract infection with dehydration, due to poor fluid intake.

He should be given oral rehydration and started on appropriate antibiotics. This is not an uncommon scenario for an elderly individual leading a solitary life.

Q 156

A 37-year-old sculptor has a recent history of feeling dizzy when she stands. She has been feeling lethargic, malaise and an inability to concentrate. She has had a dry cough for the last six weeks. She has noticed episodes of nocturia. She is on no medication, smokes 10 cigarettes a day and drinks social amounts. She has no significant medical history.

On examination, she is tanned and the skin turgor is reduced. There are no skin lesions. The pulse is 94/min, regular and her blood pressure is 120/70 mmHg and 90/50 mmHg standing. Her chest is clear. There is no abnormality in the abdomen and no specific abnormalities of the central nervous system.

- Sodium – 138 mmol/L
- Potassium – 4.5 mmol/L
- Urea – 19 mmol/L
- Creatinine –135 µmol/L
- Calcium (corrected) – 2.87 mmol/L
- Glucose – 6.2 mmol/L
- Hb –14.7 g/dl
- WBC – 12.5 x 10^9/L (85% neutrophils)
- Platelets – 297 x 10^9/L
- Chest X-ray – No abnormalities ?

- Urine dip test – No abnormalities
- Urine creatinine – 3 mmol/L
- Creatinine clearance – 68 ml/min
- Osmolarity – 320 osm/kg water
- TSH – 3 MU/L
- ADH – High normal.

A. WHAT IS THE DIAGNOSIS?

ANS: This patient has sarcoidosis with nephrogenic diabetes insipidus. The patient should undergo a chest X-ray; and the SACE level should be measured. This patient should be given steroids and adequate hydration.

The etiology of sarcoidosis is unknown. Infectious and non-infectious agents have been implicated, but no specific culprit has been found. The current evidence is consistent with the concept that the disease results from an exaggerated cellular immune response (acquired, inherited or both) to a set of antigens or self-antigens. It is more common in females and cases of sarcoidosis have been reported in all the major races, and the disease is found worldwide. Unlike many diseases in which the lung is involved, sarcoidosis favours non-smoker. Sarcoidosis causes nephrogenic diabetes insipidus by causing tubular intersitial renal disease.

Other conditions, where there may be nephrogenic diabetes insipidus due to tubular renal disease, are pylonephritis, analgesic nephropathy, mutiple myecloma, amyloidosis, obstructive uropathy, hypercalcaemia, hypokalaemic nephropathy, Sjogrens syndrome, sickle-cell anaemia and renal transplantation. The chest X-rays are almost always abnormal in sarcoidosis. There are three classic X-ray patterns in pulmonary sarcoidosis. Type I is characterised by biliteral hilar adenopathy with no parenchymal involvement. Type II is bilateral hilar adenopathy with diffuse parenchymal changes and Type III is diffuse parenchymal changes without hilar adenopathy. The Type III pattern is split into two categories with films that show fibrosis and upper lobe retraction classified separately. Although patients with type IV tend to have the acute or subacute, reversible form of the disease, while those with type II and III often have the chronic progressive disease, these patterns do not represent consecutive stages of sarcoidosis. Thus, except for epidemiological purposes, this X-ray categorisation is mostly of historical interest. The hilar adenopathy is almost always bilateral, but unilateral node enlargement can be seen. Nodes are also commonly seen in the paratracheal zone.

The diffuse parenchymal changes are typically reticulonodular infiltrates, but acini pattern may also be observed. Nodules similar to that of metastases are not uncommon. When there is massive fibrosis, the hilar are pulled upwards and there are conglomerate masses in the mid-zone. Some of the unusual chest X-ray findings in sarcoidosis include egg-shell calcification of the hilar nodes, pleural effusion, cavitations, atelectasis, pulmonary hypertension, and pneumothorax. The lung function in sarcoidosis is typical of interstitial lung disease and includes a decreased lung volume and diffusion capacity, with a normal ratio of the forced expiratory volume in 1 second to the forced vital capacity (FEV1/FVC). There may be evidence of air flow limitation. There is usually mild hypoxaemia and a mild compensated hypocarbia. The gallium 67 lung scan is usually abnormal, demonstrating a pattern of diffuse uptake; if present, extra nodes are detected as an inflammation in a number of extrathoracic sites that usually have no clinical importance.

Angiotensin converting enzymes is elevated in two-thirds of patients with sarcoidosis, but this is not diagnostic . An elevated 24-hour urine calcium level is consistent, but not specific for the disease.

B. WHAT IS THE CAUSE OF THE CALCIUM LEVEL?

ANS: The hypercalcaemia is due to a postulated increased synthesis of 1,25-dihydroxy vitamin D2 in the macrophage or other cells associated with granulomatous deposits. The level of vitamin D is further stimulated by exposure to light (natural or home solar lamp) as evident in her tanned skin.

There is a positive correlation between 25-(OH) D level (reflecting vitamin D intake), and the circulating concentration of 1,25-(OH) 2 D. Macrophages obtained from granulomatous tissues from patients with sarcoidosis form 1-25 (OH) 2 D at an increased rate when 25 (OH) D is provided as a substrate.

Q 157

A 28-year-old forestry expert has a 1-year history of painless left testicular swelling. Examination is normal and he has no lymphadenopathy. The routine baseline haematological and biochemical indices, as well as the chest X-ray and the abdominal MRI scan, are normal. The mass is not translucent and a seminoma is confirmed on orchidectomy. A course of chemotherapy was started.

Three weeks later, he complains of nausea, anorexia and a sense of pins and needles in his fingers. His wife also complains he is hard of hearing and has to turn the television volume to the full in order to hear. He has lost three kg in weight and his blood pressure is 130/80 mmHg lying and 116/58 mmHg standing. While the cuff was inflated, he developed carpopedal spasm.

Results:
- Sodium – 135 mmol/L
- Potassium – 5.1 mmol/L
- Bicarbonate – 22 mmol/L
- Urea –18 mmol/L
- Creatinine – 160 µmol/L
- Albumin – 35 g/L
- Calcium (corrected) – 2.4 mmol/L
- Urine – No protein, blood sediment or growth.

A. WHAT IS THE DIAGNOSIS?
ANS: This patient has hypomagnesaemia secondary to cisplatin therapy administered for his testicular neoplasm, which caused a carpopedal spasm.

Apart from cisplatin, aminoglycosides, diuretics and cyclosporin can also cause magnesium wasting in the urine. Cisplatin, a platinum compound, and carboplatin are the only heavy metals approved for use as anti-tumour agents. They are not true alkalising agents and they do covalently cross-link with DNA.

Cytotoxicity is determined by the balance between cellular enzymes repair or damaged DNA and the extent of the DNA cross link. Cisplatin produces nephrotoxicity and is toxic to both the proximal and the distal tubular epithelial cells. Nausea and vomiting may, at times, be severe and protracted in patients receiving cisplatin. Sensory neuropathy and high frequency hearing loss after several cycles of therapy are not uncommon.

Cisplatin has significant activity in testicular, ovarian, bladder, head, neck and lung cancers. Carboplatin is a cisplatin analogue that has less nephrotoxicity, is less emetogenic, less ototoxic, but more myelosuppressive. Most patients treated with cisplatin develop hypomagnesaemia that is severe; hypokalaemia is less common. Renal tubular mitochondria injury may be responsible for this scenario. Even after cisplatin is withdrawn, the renal defect may persist for months, years or for life.

Interestingly, calcitriol may enhance magnesium wasting in patients with cisplatin nephrotoxicity, who are also hypomagnesaemic and hypocalcaemic. Also, hypercholesterolaemia is found in a substantial percentage of cured patients years following completion of cisplatin-containing therapy.

Q 158

A 25-year-old tank gunner, a veteran of Desert Storm, undergoes an intravenous pentagastrin test. After an overnight fast, the basal gastric acid secretion is 1.1 mmol (normal is between 5–10) hydrogen H+/hour. Pantagastrin at 6 microgram/Kg is given and a sample is collected every 15 minutes.

SAMPLE	pH
1	3.9 (NORMALLY LESS THAN 2)
2	3.7
3	3.6
4	3.8

A. WHAT IS THE DIAGNOSIS?
ANS: This patient has hypoacidity due to atrophic gastritis.

B. WHAT ARE THE POSSIBLE CAUSES OF THIS CONDITION?
ANS: It can be due to surgical vagotomy, auto-immunity, and infection with helicobacter pylori.

Q 159

A 15-year-old girl has been regularly treated for intestinal Crohn's disease. The disease has been in remission.

Results:
- Hb – 9.2 g/dl
- Reticulocytes – 5.8%
- Blood film – Fragmented red cells. Heinz bodies which are seen after incubation of blood for 48 hours.

A. WHAT IS THE DIAGNOSIS?
ANS: This patient has haemolytic anaemia due to sulfasalsazine toxicity. Haemolytic anaemia caused by sulfasalazine toxicity is due to G-6-P-D deficiency.

A 78-year-old cook has had persistent ascites for the last four months.
On examination, she appears overweight and a pericardial effusion is detected on echocardiagraphy.

Results:
- Sodium – 125 mmol/L
- Cholesterol – 8.3 mmol/L
- CPK – 446 IU/L
- MCV – 110 fl

A. WHAT IS THE DIAGNOSIS?
ANS: This patient has hypothyroidism.
Hypothyroid patients have frequent muscle complaints, but weakness is only present in one third. It is predominantly proximal in nature and there may be muscle cramps, pain and stiffness. The so called myotonoid features, characterised by slow muscle contractions and relaxation, occurs in one-quarter of patients and are often accompanied by myxoedema (local contraction produced by tapping or pinching the muscle).
The serum CK levels are often elevated (up to 10 times normal) even with minimal clinical evidence of muscle disease.

Q 161

A 75-year-old matron of an obstetrical unit has lower sternal dysphagia and a sense of weakness for the last six months. She has been working very hard and has noticed some discolouration on the back of her hands. She was reassured by her colleagues that this was probably due to an allergic reaction to the Hibiscrub which she is using. She sent her blood for analysis.

Results:
- Hb – 11.2 g/dl
- MCV – 83 fl
- Platelets – 656 x 10⁹/L
- ESR – 45 mm/hour
- CPK – 780 IU/L
- AST – 130 IU/L

A. What is this patient's diagnosis?
Ans: This patient has dermatomyositis with oesophageal cancer.

The discolouration on the back of her hands is called Gottran's papules. The diagnosis may be confirmed by EMG muscle biopsy and a barium swallow.

Q 162

A 21-year-old British nanny undergoes a gastric acid study for dyspepsia. She also complains of intermittent diarrhoea. The girl appears to be psychologically disturbed at times and this has caused great concern to the parents. She has no familial history of a similar complaint.

The basal acid output is 17mmol/hour (normal range is 5–10). The peak acid output is 24 mmol/hour (normal range is less than 50). Her serum calcium level is 2.35 mmol/L.

A. What is this patient's most likely diagnosis?
Ans: This patient has the Zollinger-Ellison (Z-E) syndrome with vitamin B12 malabsorption.

Vitamin B12 malabsoption, which is not corrected by intrinsic factor, is seen in some patients with Z-E syndrome. Although gastric secretion of intrinsic factor appears normal, the reduced pH in the gut interferes with the intrinsic mediated vitamin B12 absorption. This can be corrected by neutralisation of the intestinal content.

The exact mechanisms in which the low pH in the gut interferes with intrinsic factor action are unknown. The diarrhoea is due to the outpouring of large amounts of hydrochloric acid and can be reduced or eliminated by aspiration of gastric juice. The diarrhoea is not strictly secretory, but is due in part to the maldigestion of fat, caused by inactivation of pancreatic lipase and precipitation of bile salts and low pH.

Cobalamine malabsorption occurs, but this abnormality is invariably mild and never causes clinical cobalamine deficiency. In 1955, Zollinger and Ellison reported the association between peptic ulcer and gastrin-secreting tumours of the pancreas. The elevated gastrin level leads to hypersecretion of acid and consequent to duodenal and jejunal ulcers.

Ninety percent of gastrinomas are found within an anatomical triangle called the gastrinoma triangle. This comprises of
i)   The junction of the cystic and the common bile duct superiorly.
ii) The junction of the 2nd and 3rd portion of the duodenum inferiorly.
iii) The junction of the pancreatic body and neck medially.

In up to 60% of patients with Z-E syndrome, gastrinoma is a component of the MEN I syndrome, an autosomal dominant disorder with a high degree of penetration and a great variable expressitivity.

About two-thirds of gastrinomas are histologically or biologically malignant. Detection of hypergastric secretion is important when the Z-E syndrome is suspected. Since patients with benign gastric ulcers secrete some acid, pentagastrin fast achlohydria in a patient with gastric ulcer is almost always associated with a malignancy. As the basal acid output is relatively high and the peak acid output does not elevate significantly with pentagastrin, this suggests an autonomous neoplasm. One may perform a MRI or a CT scan of the abdomen, and measure the gastric level. Radiologic and endoscopic examination may reveal increased gastric fluid and thickened rugae.

The technique for measuring gastric output is to use a radio-opaque gastric tube which is passed so that its tip is located in the lowest portion of the stomach. With the patient reclining or semi-recumbent on the left side, the tube position is verified by fluoroscopy. The gastric contents are aspirated and discarded. Secretions are then collected in four consecutive 15-minute intervals to determine the one-hour basal acid secretion volume and acid concentration (titrated with sodium hydroxide to pH 7 or calculated by formula from the pH of the aspirated gastric juice). Gastric output is expressed in mmol/hour. Maximal gastric output may be stimulated by histamine, betazole (histalog) and pentagastrin.

B. How would you treat this patient?
Ans: The treatment is directed at the sequelae of excess gastrin secretion and the tumour itself. Omeprozole has decreased the need of surgery for these patients. The rare patients who fail to response to medical therapy should be treated surgically. There is no evidence that tumour progression is influenced by gastrectomy.

In patients with coexisting hyperparathyroidism, parathyroid resection should be performed before a decision about gastric surgery is needed, since the resolution of hypercalcaemia may permit better medical control of gastric acid secretion.

C. What are the other uses of gastric acid secretory studies?
Ans: Apart from the Zollinger-Ellison syndrome or atropic gastritis, it may also be used for the determination of the completeness of vagotomy.

Suspected gastric cancer is better diagnosed directly through a gastroscope and biopsy than indirectly with acid secretory studies (achlohydria). This study should not be obtained for routine diagnosis of uncomplicated duodenal ulcer. Acid studies are not useful in determining the type of surgery for duodenal ulcer.

Q 163

A 62-year-old light house keeper has had pale offensive stools for the last six months and has lost 10 kg in weight. Fifteen years ago, he underwent emergency surgery for a bleeding gastric ulcer. He attended a conference of oceanographers one year ago. During the time in Russia, he traveled extensively and visited various parts of the Ukraine and St. Petersburg. He spends most of the time reading, but he finds it difficult now as his vision seems to be falling.

- Hb – 9.9 g/dl
- MCV – 84 fl
- WBC – 4.1 x 10⁹/L
- Platelets – 450 x 10⁹/L
- Sodium – 128 mmol/L
- Potassium – 2.8 mmol/L
- Calcium – 2.02 mmol/L
- Phosphate – 0.67 mmol/L
- Albumin – 28 g/L
- AST – 15 IU/L
- Alkaline phosphatase – 349 IU/L
- Vitamin B12 –142 nanograms/L
- Serum folate – 4.5 µgrams/L
- Red cell folate – 610 micrograms/L
- Fecal fat collection – 18 g/day

A. WHAT IS THE DIAGNOSIS?

ANS: This patient has post-gastrectomy malabsorption and the blind loop syndrome.

In the blind loop syndrome, the bacteria takes up vitamin B12 and impairs the absorption of B12. The serum folate produced by the bacteria explains its elevated level in this patient. Although the cause of cobalamine deficiency after partial gastrectotomy may be an intestinal overgrowth of bacteria, it does not always respond to antibiotics.

Malabsorption syndrome has been documented frequently in patients after subtotal gastrectomy. Steatorrhoea is more common with Billroth type II than Billroth type I anastomosis. Usually the fat loss is minimal, ranging from 7–10 grams/24 hours. Patients with gross steatorrhea usually have impaired intraluminal fat digestion. This may be due to the decreased stimulus for the release of secretin and cholecystokinin (pancreozymin) from the duodenum (as with the Billroth II anastomosis, the duodenum is bypassed) and results in a depressed pancreatic enzyme response. There may be inadequate mixing of pancreatic enzymes and bile salts secreted into the duodenum with the gastric content entering the jejunum. There may be stasis of intestinal contents in the afferent loop, resulting in abnormal bacteria proliferation in the proximal small bowel, as in this case.

The presence of maldigestion may lead to protein depletion which in turn impairs pancreatic function. The loss of the reservoir function of the stomach results in increased intestinal transit time.

B. WHAT OTHER DIAGNOSIS WOULD YOU CONSIDER?
ANS: One should also consider the possibility of coeliac disease, giardiasis and primary intestinal lymphoma.

The usual stigmata of generalised lymphoma are frequently absent, but there is hepatomegaly and splenomegaly palpable. Malabsorption in intestinal lymphoma is due to diffuse involvement of the small intestinal mucosa, bowel wall with lymphatic obstruction, localised stenosis with stasis of intestinal contents, and bacteria overgrowth. It is difficult to distinguish coeliac sprue from intestinal lymphoma. There is evidence that suggests that lymphoma may develop as a late complication of coeliac sprue. The course of intestinal lymphoma ranges from four months to four years from the onset of symptoms.

Perforation bleeding and intestinal obstruction are possible terminal complications. There is inadequate evidence to determine whether radiation therapy, chemotherapy or surgical resection alters the natural history of this disease.

Q 164

A 35-year-old gypsy dancer, who was admitted for an acute unilateral parotitis, suddenly complains of severe abdominal pain.

On clinical examination, she appears distressed, anxious and has a low grade fever. Her BP is 110/60 mmHg and there are erythematous skin nodules over her chest. On auscultation, she has bibasal crackles and left-sided pleural effusion. The ECG shows ST segments and T-wave abnormality in the lateral leads. Soon after the ECG was taken, she is suddenly blind in the right eye.

Results:
• Sodium – 125 mmols/L
• Potassium – 5.8 mmols/L
• Albumin – 26 g/L
• Calcium – 1.68 mmols/L
• AST – 213 IU/L
• Urea – 16.8 mmols/L

A. WHAT IS THE LIKELY DIAGNOSIS?

ANS: This patient has acute pancreatitis induced by mumps.

In acute pancreatitis the serum amylase is usually elevated within 24 hours and remains so for 1–3 days. The total amylase level returns more rapidly than pancreatic isoamylase. In patients seen after the 1st day, the pancreatic isoamylase level is more sensitive of pancreatitis than the total serum amylase levels. The serum trypsinogen is helpful in an equivocal isoamylase level. This enzyme is secreted specifically by the pancreas. A normal serum trypsinogen level in a patient with minimal elevation of serum amylase rules out acute pancreatitis. Lipase may now be the single best enzyme for the diagnosis of acute pancreatitis. The newer lipase assays have co-lipase as a co-factor and are fully automated. Many hospital laboratories are now using Ekthachem technique because it is rapid and contains the appropriate substrates. Reports have demonstrated poor specificity with this technique, i.e. patients with non-pancreatic disorders having elevated lipase levels.

The erythematous skin nodules present are due to subcutaneous fat necrosis. Purtscher's retinopathy, a relatively unusual complication refers to the sudden severe loss of vision in a patient with acute pancreatitis and is characterised by peculiar fundoscopic appearance of cotton wool spots and haemorrhage confined to an area limited by the optic disc and macular. The pathology is due to posterior renal artery occlusion with aggregated granulocytes. A contrast enhanced dynamic CT (CECT) scan provides valuable information for the prognosis and the severity of acute pancreatitis. CECT allows estimation of the presence and extent of pancreatic necrosis.

Q 165

A 26-year-old artist is admitted with early morning headache, vomiting and deterioration in her vision which interferes with her painting. She is currently on medication for manic-depressive psychosis and has a history of an attempted suicide four years ago. She does not have any clinical symptoms suggesting any dysfunction of the thyroid organ and is well hydrated.

On examination, she appears slightly overweight, visual acuity is slightly reduced and there is mild peripheral constriction of visual fields and bilateral papilloedema is noted.

A. WHAT IS THE DIAGNOSIS?
ANS: This patient has lithium-induced benign intracranial hypertension.

B. WHAT ARE THE OTHER CAUSES OF THIS DISORDER?
ANS: The other conditions which may predisposed to benign intracranial hypertension are endocrinological dysfunctions such as hypothyroidism, hyperthyroidism, hypoparathyroidism, adrenal insufficiency, excess of endogenous and exogenous adreno-corticoids.

The other association occurs with sarcoidosis and SLE. Some drugs have been implicated including Vitamin A, outdated tetracycline, nalidixic acid, nitrofurantoin, sulphonamides, indomethacin and phenytoin.

C. HOW WOULD YOU CONFIRM THE DIAGNOSIS?
ANS: This is confirmed by the exclusion of an intracranial mass lesion or meningeal cancer.

In the presence of a normal or small ventricular system on CT or MRI scan, a lumbar puncture carries no risk for brain herniation. Cerebrospinal fluid is invariable under increased pressure.

Treatment is aimed at preventing visual deterioration by repetitive lumbar puncture and by cessation of lithium. The patient should be put on carbamazepine instead. Patients refractory to this may benefit from acetazolamide or a short term glucocorticoid therapy. Lumboperitoneal shunting, surgical subtemporal decompression or optic nerve sheath fenestration is only used for patients with progressive visual impairment who have failed to improve with aggressive therapy.

Q 166

A 37-year-old Japanese sushi chef has been asked by her employer to seek medical advice as one of her eyes appears to be enlarging. She has obvious left-sided proptosis and complains of seeing double for the last three weeks, but has no other symptoms of hyperthyroidism.

The clinical examination reveals she is clinically euthyroid. She has no significant medical history, except for an appendectomy six years ago.

A. What is the diagnosis?

Ans: This patient has euthyroid Grave's disease.

Ophthalmoplegia in the absence of infiltrative manifestation can be confused with that which occurs in diabetes mellitus, myasthenia gravis and myopathies. When there is an uncertainty of ophthalmopathy, the demonstration of significant titres of TSI, TBII, of an abnormal TRH stimulation or thyroid suppression, suggests the cause is Grave's disease, though not all patients with euthyroid Grave's disease demonstrate abnormal responses.

In such cases, ultrasonography, MRI or CT tomography of the orbit is useful in demonstrating characteristic thickening of the extra-ocular muscle.

Q 167

A 72-year-old retired air-force general notices he has a tendency to bump into objects on his right. For the last three weeks his friends have noted confusion, apathy, drowsiness and a deterioration in his intellect. He has difficulty in dressing. These symptoms have caused grave concern to his family. His mistress notices he has a tendency to drag his right limb.

On examination, he is drowsy, disoriented and confused. His left pupil is larger, but reactive. The rest of the cranial examination appears clinically normal. Fundoscopy and visual field testing do not reveal any abnormality. He has an intermittent ability to follow oral instructions. The tone in his right arm and leg are increased. The sensation is intact, but there is a right sensory inattention and he has idiomotor apraxia.

A. What is the most likely diagnosis?

Ans: This patient has a left subdural haematoma.

The dilated pupil is due to the tentorial herniation and the involvement of the 3rd nerve. The diagnosis is readily confirmed by CT scan and the therapeutic management is early surgical management.

B. What other diagnosis would you consider?

Ans: A left glioma and a cerebrovascular accident.

Q 168

A 42-year-old kayaker is brought to casualty with headache and drowsiness. Three hours prior to admission, he had developed a headache and vomited several times. He had become unconscious for a few minutes. Upon gaining consciousness, he complains of seeing double in all directions of gaze. He is on amlodipine for hypertension.

On examination, he is febrile and very drowsy. His pupils are small, but reactive. There is nystagmus in all directions of gaze. He is dysarthric and the finger-nose co-ordination is poor, particularly on the left. The tone, power and sensation are normal, but reflexes are bilaterally brisk.

A. WHAT IS THE MOST LIKELY DIAGNOSIS?

ANS: This patient has a cerebellar haematoma. This is readily confirmed on CT scan.

Surgical therapy of acute cerebellar haemorrhage is nearly always recommended as it prevents secondary brainstem compression and provides an excellent prognosis for recovery. If this patient is alert without focal brainstem sign and the cerebellar haematoma is small (on CT scan), surgical removal may not be indicated.

Mannitol and osmotic agents reduce intracranial pressure that has been elevated by the volume of haematoma and oedema. Glucocorticoids are of uncertain value in controlling the oedema from intracerebral haematoma. Excessive hypo and hypertension should be avoided.

Q 169

A 26-year-old student of marine biology, who specialises in the behaviour of dolphins, is referred to the university physician with complaints of pins and needles in her lower limbs and feet, with a feeling of a bandage being tightly wrapped around her knees. The symptoms developed over the last three weeks. She had noticed a blurring of vision. She has changed her glasses several times during the last few months, but her vision has not improved. Her lecturers have noticed that she has had a change in personality with impaired judgement and inappropriate jocularity. She has noticed an increased frequency and urgency of micturation, and described an episode of dizziness lasting three weeks which resolved spontaneously.

On examination, there are no abnormal signs in the cranial nerves. She has a tattoo on her left arm and an examination of her lower limbs show increased tone with weakness in knee flexion and dorsiflexion, and bilateral increased tendon reflexes with a positive Babinski's sign. Sensation is impaired and there is a decreased vibration and joint position sense in the lower limbs. A sensory level to light touch was found at T_4. Physical examination does not reveal any other abnormality apart from an old healed appendicectomy scar.

A. WHAT IS THE PROBABLE DIAGNOSIS?

ANS: This patient has multiple sclerosis (MS) with the involvement of the spinal cord at the T_4 level.

Multiple sclerosis derived its name from the multiple scarred areas visible on macroscopic examination of the brain. These plaques are well-demarcated pink or grey areas easily distinguished from the white matter. The correlation of plaque numbers and size with clinical symptoms is poor. It is paradoxical that in an extensive plaque burden may be associated with only mild symptoms, or conversely, minor pathological findings may be present in some severely disabled individuals. Ectopic impulses generation or cross talk might give rise to Lhermitt's syndrome, paroxysmal symptoms of parasthesia. Evidence for an environmental effect on multiple sclerosis is postulated from epidemics that have occurred, e.g. the cluster of cases of multiple sclerosis that occurred in the Faroe Islands off the coast of Denmark during the Second World War.

The involvement of the spinal cord at a specific level is diagnostic because it distinguishes the sensory attack from the peripheral neuropathies due to Gullian-Barré syndrome, mononeuropathy multiplex or toxins. The visual blurring may be due to optic neuritis secondary to the plaque which is associated with this condition. Cognitive dysfunction is common in cases of advanced multiple sclerosis, but may also occur in early or mild disease. Rarely are cognitive symptoms the initial manifestation of the disease. Memory loss is the most important cognitive loss in multiple sclerosis.

In one study that assessed function 25 years after the initial diagnosis of multiple sclerosis, 1/4 of the cases remained capable of work and 1/2 were still ambulatory. Other studies have revealed a less favourable prognosis. In general the longer that a population is followed, the smaller is the population of patients with mild disease. SLE may, on rare occasions, mimic multiple sclerosis. Other signs of SLE are usually present including an elevated ESR, autoantibodies and evidence of systemic disease.Neurological involvement in SLE may simulate optic neuritis or transverse myelitis. The myelopathy in SLE may be acute or chronic, or may be due to vasculitis or infarction rather than to primary demyelination.

A 3-year trial of beta-interferon therapy in relapsing remitting multiple sclerosis indicated that this treatment lessened the frequency of the attacks by 30% and reduced disease activity by 80% as assessed by MRI. Patients who enrolled for this trial were ambulatory without support and had experienced at least two MS attacks in the previous two years. This sub-group of patients should therefore be considered as candidates for subcutaneously administered beta-interferon which was approved for use in 1993. It is uncertain whether the beneficial effects of beta-interferon are due to its antiviral or its immunosuppressive properties.

ACKNOWLEDGEMENTS

The author wishes firstly to thank H.E. Tsem Tulku Rinpoche for his blessings to publish this book and for his Foreword. I first met Rinpoche one and a half years ago. Since that moment, I have felt that Rinpoche has always been close and protective to my family and me in many inexplicable ways and guided my practice in the art and science of medicine. The brilliant Professor of Cardiology, Desmond G. Julian once wrote that half of what we teach of medicine is wrong but we don't know which half. He was describing the flow of compassion, wisdom, inspiration and intuition, when we have faith in making the right decision in healing our patients. I have faith in Rinpoche in guiding me to choose the right from wrong in all aspects of my life and I know that all that is good in me comes from Rinpoche.

I also wish to give special thanks to my dear wife, Dr. Ming Hui Ying, whose advice and assistance throughout the writing of this book has been invaluable.

Finally, I would also like to thank the following individuals for their contribution and efforts in producing this Book (in alphabetical order)

- Su-Lin Chee
- Jeannie Chen
- Kam-Choon Goh
- Jamie Khoo
- Susan Lim
- Joan Foo Mahony
- Voon-Chin Ngeow
- Deborah Pereira
- Li-Kim Phng
- Sharon Saw
- Kah-Hoong Thor
- Yoke-Fui Yap

INDEX

autosomal, 14, 46, 48, 71, 77, 85, 94, 109, 169, 190, 202, 216
axilla, axillary, 20, 45, 107, 163, 182, 208
azotemia, 17, 25, 127, 179

B

Babinski's sign, 224
bacteria, 32, 80, 82, 90, 97, 98, 116, 118, 128, 149, 164, 199, 218, 219
Barter's syndrome, 189, 190
Bell's palsy, 108
Berger's disease, 200
beri-beri, 27, 60, 153
beta, 22, 75, 80, 105, 114, 180, 189, 190, 191, 225
bile, 24, 28, 29, 82, 98, 166, 199, 201, 216, 218
bilirubin, 24, 26, 28, 31, 52, 53, 63, 65, 79, 88, 89, 103, 129, 134, 140, 146, 163, 164, 166, 178, 179, 194
biopsy (non-liver), 35, 44, 45, 46, 50, 58, 61, 74, 81, 86, 97, 107, 128, 147, 150, 152, 175, 188, 199, 200, 207, 208, 215, 217
bladder, 59, 102, 130, 139, 140, 166, 169, 175, 198, 199, 206, 212
blind loop, 82, 218
blood culture, 37, 39, 43, 44, 71, 123, 135, 148, 167, 185, 206
blood pressure, 14, 18, 20, 27, 29, 31, 36, 38, 40, 42, 54, 60, 63, 68, 71, 74, 75, 79, 85, 87, 89, 119, 120, 122, 125, 127, 128, 129, 167, 169, 170, 172, 182, 190, 193, 205, 207, 208, 209, 212
bone, 15, 42, 44, 45, 89, 132, 134, 135, 161, 162, 165, 166, 188, 189, 206

bone marrow, 44, 45, 89, 92, 132, 134, 135, 161, 162, 165, 206
botulism, 70, 130, 131
bowel, 14, 52, 80, 81, 83, 94, 107, 135, 180, 182, 202, 218, 219
BP (blood pressure), 12, 13, 16, 19, 21, 56, 83, 107, 109, 111, 112, 115, 117, 135, 140, 180, 184, 189, 191, 196, 198, 219
bradycardia, 20, 119, 120
bronchi, 21, 22, 55, 58, 117, 132, 135
Brown-Sequard syndrome, 140
brucellosis, 43, 44
Brugada Syndrome, 60
Buerger's disease, 128, 132
Bulimia, 153
bypass, 27, 69, 96, 98

C

caesarian section, 20, 130, 149
calcification, 19, 189, 211
cancer, 52, 91, 112, 115, 175, 177, 213, 215, 217, 221
carcinoma, 33, 52, 66, 70, 90, 121, 140, 203
cardiomyopathy, 27, 51, 79, 119
Caroli's disease, 166
carotid, 56, 68, 69, 119, 120, 154, 155, 157, 159
catheter, catheterisation, 14, 17, 105, 182, 206, 207
central nervous system, 39, 41, 45, 67, 86, 128, 194, 205, 209
cerebellopontine myelinolysis (CPM), 81
cerebral, 14, 41, 43, 56, 65, 68, 69, 91, 126, 152, 158, 159, 170, 176, 177, 187, 197, 221, 223

LaVergne, TN USA
23 August 2009
155651LV00002B/3/P